SERENITY THEFT

SERENITY THEFT

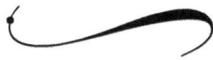

TWELVE SIMPLE WAYS TO STOP
STRESS AND RESTORE CALM

Wendy Lee Jaques

ISBN-13: 9780692515914
ISBN-10: 0692515917
Library of Congress Control Number: 2015916383
Wendy Lee Jaques, Houston, TX

Half of me is filled with bursting words and half of me is painfully shy. I crave solitude yet also crave people. I want to put life and love into everything yet also nurture myself with care and go gently. I want to live within the rush of primal intuitive decision, yet also wish to sit and contemplate. This is the messiness of life—that we all carry multitudes, so must sit with the shifts. We are complicated creatures and the balance comes from that understanding. Be okay with the flow. Be water. Flexible and soft. Subtly powerful and open. Wild and serene, able to carry and accept all changes yet still led by the pull of steady tides. It is enough.

—Victoria Erickson

CONTENTS

PREFACE

JUNE 15, 2001, was one of the happiest days of my life. It was the day my daughter, Lily, was born. My husband, Steve, and I had been married for seven years, and we had been trying to have a baby for four. When we first met Lily and took her home, it seemed life was complete. But our idyllic time as parents did not last long—especially for me. Having a newborn baby is stressful, even in the best of times. The September 11 attacks happened when Lily was just three months old. I was devastated, like the rest of the country, and I had no idea what this meant for the world my daughter would grow up in. I cried for a week.

Just as I began to feel a little better, our family faced another tragedy. On September 26, Steve and I received the news that Steve's brother had passed away suddenly of a heart attack, leaving behind his wife and two small children. A few days later, we were on a plane from Houston, Texas, to Vancouver, British Columbia, Canada, to attend the funeral, support our family, and mourn our loss.

The following month, November, we found ourselves headed on another unexpected trip, this time to Clarkston, Washington. My grandmother was turning eighty-six, and she was in failing health. We did not know if she was going to be around much longer, and we wanted to celebrate her birthday for what would likely be the last time.

After that, I was fully exhausted, both emotionally and physically. Traveling while breast-feeding and caring for my infant child was draining and stressful, and I was looking forward to the chance to rest at home with my family during the Christmas season. Unfortunately, we had planned a family trip over the holiday. It was the only vacation we had planned for that year. We had planned it months in advance, long before all the other unexpected events. I did not want to go, but everyone reassured me there would be lots of help with the baby, which would allow me time to rest. Against my better judgment, I got on a plane bound for Canada to spend Christmas with my in-laws.

On the way there, my thoughts soured. I did not want anyone's help. I just wanted to be at home with my husband and my baby. I wanted to sleep, eat, and rest. I know my family meant well and had the best of intentions. However, at that point I did not care how well intentioned they were; my and Lily's needs were all that mattered. Upon our return home, I was so tired that it was beginning to really take a toll on my mind and body. I was extremely stressed out, my anxiety was through the roof, and I began experiencing severe postpartum depression. A few days after Christmas, we returned home to Houston. It was 2002, and on New Year's Day, I had a complete meltdown. I was beyond exhausted, and I felt like I was going mad. I ended up in the corner of my living room, curled up in the fetal position, crying hysterically, rocking back and forth. I did not know what was happening to me. Over the next few days, I grew very ill. I developed a fever and could hardly get out of bed. My temperature hovered around 102 degrees for three days; all the while I tried to breast-feed my baby girl. At about eleven o'clock on the third night of my illness, I drove myself to the ER; Steve stayed with Lily. When I arrived, there were others in the ER, but the nurses took me right back once they learned I had had such a high fever for three days. I knew from my days working as an EMT that, according to the rules of triage, I was in a bad situation. They did a chest X-ray and discovered a spot on my lung, indicating pneumonia. They informed me that I needed to start taking a heavy-duty antibiotic right away, and I would have to stop breast-feeding my six-month-old daughter. I was devastated. This moment was the turning point for me.

Someone had come in and stolen the life I had envisioned for myself and left me with a life I didn't want. But I didn't know how to change that, or so I thought. Our bodies are intuitive. We just have to learn how to listen with intention.

Something primal welled up inside of me. I straight up told the doctors that I was not going to stop breast-feeding my child, and they were going to have to find something else that I could take. It's amazing what a little bit of coercion can do. They found an antibiotic that was considered safe for nursing mothers and infants. Of course, I was terrified on many levels. Was this medication going to harm my child? Being so ill, was my body going to produce enough milk for my child to thrive? Was I going to die? Amazingly, it did get better; I didn't die, and I produced plenty of milk.

As my health began to improve, I was focused on doing everything I could to get better, so I could be the very best mom I could be to my daughter. As tired and depleted as I felt, I had an overwhelming drive to fight my way back to optimal health. Little did I know the long journey ahead of me. For the next several months, I suffered chronic yeast infections, chronic bronchial infections, sinus infections, chronic fatigue, severe weight loss, and alternating bouts of constipation and diarrhea. My weight went down to 123 pounds. At five feet eleven inches, I was so unhealthy and depleted that my ability to be the healthy, vibrant mom and wife that I wanted and needed to be became compromised. I was doing all the right things, eating well, exercising, resting, trying to reduce my stress, but my body was just not absorbing the nutrients in my food. My face was gaunt, my skin was pale and pasty, my hair was falling out, and I felt that the essence of the person I was, was slipping away. The light of my spirit was growing dim. I literally felt like I was dying.

When I followed up with my primary care physician, the diagnosis was profound. He said I was depressed and had chronic fatigue syndrome. I already knew that! What I wanted was some support—a plan to get my health back. So far, that was something the doctors around me could not provide. I was so frustrated. I left with a few prescriptions, which I never filled, and knew in my mind there had to be another way.

My counselor at the time referred me to a naturopath—a homeopathic doctor. Two to three times a week for the next several months, I would drive twenty-five miles each way to see this doctor, who I believed would lead me back to my old self. I put my full faith in him and saw him to be my only option. I was desperate, not in a good position to make such important decisions about my health. The procedures, tests, and treatment plans began to feel more like some strange scientific experiment in the worst sci-fi B movie ever, rather than something that was really going to help me. This doctor prescribed massive amounts of supplements. Each week, he would add another one or tell me to stop taking one he had just prescribed. He had his own little pharmacy there in his office, and he even gave me an alternative medicine that turned out to be expired. I know this sounds crazy and foolish, but I wanted to believe that this man would help me regain my health. Besides that, I trusted the counselor who had referred me to him.

My health crisis was new to me. I knew that I didn't understand how it should be treated, so I just kept showing up, hoping something the doctor did would help. I remember the day I went into his office to discuss my treatment plan with him. I told him I had started on a thyroid medication that my general practitioner had prescribed because the one he had given me had expired. He proceeded to berate me, telling me he couldn't help me if I was not going to be 100 percent committed to his program. He didn't want to deal with a "loose cannon." In the exam room, with my baby daughter on my lap, I was reduced to tears, completely humiliated. At that moment, I knew that would be my last appointment with him. I felt dejected, helpless, and discouraged. I thought to myself, if this is the alternative and it didn't work, what now?

When I got home, I tallied up the money I had spent on this doctor. After several months working with him, the total came to thousands of dollars, and I knew insurance wouldn't cover it. I was in despair.

I was in despair, but I was not defeated. I found another alternative medicine doctor recommended by a good friend, and this new doctor helped me begin a true healing process. My daughter was my sole motivation. I wanted to be healthy for her. I didn't want to be just a *good* mommy, I wanted to be the *best* mommy she could possibly have. I realized that for that to happen, I was going to have to dig deep—deeper than I ever had before.

This new doctor not only practiced alternative medicine but also was a Christian, unlike the previous homeopath (psychopath) who treated me. My first visit was unlike any I had experienced at a doctor's office. It was almost as if this new doctor knew me even before my first visit. It was as if every staff member had prepared for my arrival. The visit evoked that feeling you get when you walk down the freezer aisle in the grocery store and all the lights come on. Being in that office felt familiar and right. I thought to myself, this is how everyone should be treated when going to the doctor. I had renewed hope and knew I was going to get well. It took me two years to feel like myself again, and during the healing process, I learned that nobody else was going to bring me back from the brink. I had to take charge of my own body and my own health.

We have much more power in our own health and healing than we realize!

My journey taught me to be my own health advocate. I've learned how to ask myself the right questions to lead myself down the right path, not only in the area of health, but also in every area of my life. My prayer was that God would somehow use my experience to help others in a mighty way and, ultimately, it would glorify Him.

Here I am fifteen years later, answering the call to use my story to empower others to defeat disease, reclaim their health, and be the change they desire in their own lives. I am helping others realize that God has given us amazing power to grow, to change, and to heal not only ourselves but also others.

In the midst of my illness, I cried out to God, asking, "How am I supposed to do this? How am I supposed to be a good wife, a mother to my daughter, and live the fulfilling life that I've always dreamed of?" He made it so simple for me and eased my fears and anxieties. He led me to Matthew 22:36–39 (NASB):

> "Teacher, which is the great commandment in the Law?" And He said to him, "YOU SHALL LOVE THE LORD YOUR GOD WITH ALL YOUR HEART, AND WITH ALL YOUR SOUL, AND WITH ALL YOUR MIND. This is the great and foremost commandment. The second is like it, YOU SHALL LOVE YOUR NEIGHBOR AS YOURSELF."

Love God. Love others. It was as simple as that. My closest neighbor was my family. Love God and love my family. For the next year, that is what I did. This book contains the tools I gradually incorporated into my life and their healing powers. Before I knew it, I had discovered a transformative lifestyle.

INTRODUCTION

HERE'S MY DEFINITION of serenity theft: the fraudulent acquisition of a person's serenity resulting in the theft of a person's joy and happiness. The culprit? Stress.

To prevent serenity theft, experts recommend that you regularly check in with yourself and manage your stress and, in the process, destroy any unsolicited joy killers. Follow up with your stress busters daily to protect yourself from unwanted burnout, anxiety, and disease.

Consider Dr. Archibald D. Hart's assessment of one of the modern-day causes of stress: "Your mind and body were designed for camel speed. Your life is moving at the speed of a cheetah. No wonder you are stressed, anxious, and depressed." Stress, anxiety, and depression are known as S-A-D. In *The Anxiety Cure*, Dr. Hart describes the volatile relationship among these foes:

> [1]If only anxiety would stick to itself and not team up with other problems, it would be a lot easier to cope with. Anxiety always has fellow travelers. Some just go along for the ride, but others insist on getting into the act as well. So anyone struggling to overcome an anxiety problem must also learn how to deal with these freeloaders as well, especially depression. They sponge off the anxiety and make life more complicated than we would like it to be.

---

1 Archibald D. Hart, *The Anxiety Cure: You Can Find Emotional Tranquility and Wholeness* (Nashville, Tennessee: Thomas Nelson, 1999) 168

This book will teach you practices that will improve your overall health and happiness and reduce the stress in your life. I won't urge you to make big changes in your life. Actually, it is the small, simple changes we make that bring about lasting and transformative change.

Wellness comes from the health of both the mind and the body. The first step to better health is to identify what is holding you back. I don't know about you, but I have a huge fear of change, especially when I can't see or control how it will look on the other side. Quite frankly, the thought of change stresses me out! And many others feel the same way. That fear can be the biggest stumbling block to making positive change.

Ask yourself these questions to understand how to achieve the best health of your life:

- Do I constantly feel stressed, overwhelmed, and exhausted?
- Do I feel like I am on the brink of a mental or physical breakdown and don't know how to stop it from happening?
- Am I looking for a natural way to relieve anxiety and depression?
- Do I ever feel like I've disconnected from my life or am just going through the motions?
- Do I ever ask myself, "Is this as good as it gets?"
- Am I in a rut that I can't seem to break free of?
- Am I struggling to shed those extra pounds and longing to look and feel my best?
- Am I confused and frustrated with all the conflicting dietary theories, wondering which one is right for me?
- Do I dream of living an energy-filled life?

For years, these questions haunted me, until one day my body told me to sit down, shut up, and listen.

During a major health scare and the subsequent two-year recovery period, I realized the time had come to make drastic changes to my life, and I learned my body held answers for me, but my thinking was limited by fear. My body was sending me a clear and strong message that change needed to happen for my own physical and mental health, and it needed to happen now! Meanwhile, my brain feared how I would get there. I realized I had to trust my body's inner wisdom.

One thing that became very clear to me was that people often block their own paths to progress. We may not recognize this, and we may blame other people or circumstances for our failure to reach our goals or fulfill our dreams. The reality is that *nothing external* is stopping us from fulfilling our highest potential and moving toward making those positive changes we've been dreaming about. Our own thoughts and limiting beliefs are what get in our way.

Here's how it works: Your thoughts, especially those negative, nagging ones, dictate your emotions. These, in turn, influence your beliefs about what you can accomplish. Through this process, you create your own reality, which is ultimately governed by your thoughts.

Thoughts Emotions Beliefs = Your Reality

If you are dissatisfied with some aspect of your life, start turning inside to look at your own thoughts and beliefs. Consider the choices you're making and how they are serving you or holding you back. You own the key to making the necessary changes. Nobody else does. You have the power to make things happen in your life—for better and for worse. As daunting as this sounds, the bright side is that you get to choose what direction your life takes. In this book, you will find a wealth of information to help you gain control of stress and stop allowing it to control you and rob you of joy, peace, and calm. You will learn methods to help neutralize the harmful effects of stress on your mind, body, spirit, and the spaces around you. You will understand strategies and healthy coping mechanisms, including many that I have incorporated into my own life. It's time to stop the stress and restore the calm, one simple change at a time!

Today is a new day. You shall begin it serenely and with too high a spirit to be encumbered with your old nonsense.

—Ralph Waldo Emerson

CHAPTER 1

UNDERSTAND HEALTH COACHING

The conscious effort to understand your mind, body, spirit, intuitive thoughts, habits, memories, impulses etc., comes from within. It is at this reference point that healing is cultivated. It begins and continues from within. One must reach far inside to find that spark that initiates self-understanding and healing. No one can do this for you. However, we can partner with others to inspire, empower, support, and celebrate one another.

—JANNIE B., HEALTH COACH AND GRADUATE OF IIN

People do not care how much you know until they know how much you care. They usually will not remember what you said or what you did, but they will most certainly remember how you made them feel.

—WENDY LEE JAQUES

THE MOST IMPORTANT aspects of healing are the belief of the patient, the belief of the healer, and the relationship between the two. A health coach does what most doctors don't want to do, don't have time to do, and are not trained to do. Doctors are taught about disease management. Most receive less than twenty-four hours of nutritional training in all their years in medical school. It is a rare thing to find a doctor who will work with you on stress management, relationship challenges, or how to uncover the root cause of your disease processes instead of just playing a game of whack-a-mole. Many of the diseases we face are the result of stress in our lives, especially stress in our careers and relationships. This is compounded by the physical stress caused by a sedentary lifestyle and poor-quality nutrition. Our food and lifestyle choices are the foundations for our health and well-being, and they affect our ability to deal with stress. A health coach looks at the whole person and the whole life: listening, caring, and creating strategies for health, healing, and happiness. A health coach empowers his or her clients to ultimately heal themselves. A health coach listens to clients and their stories and allays their fears. If clients walk away feeling good about the relationship with their coach and about their visit, chances are they will get better in spite of the medicines they may be taking.

Western medicine is very procedural. You take the blood pressure, heart rate, and respirations. You do the blood work, EKG, and chest X-ray. You go up to the wards in the hospital. The doctor looks at the test results and presents the case the next morning. There is a place for this, and it is often a necessary part of the process, but a relationship with the patient is not encouraged. In many other countries, health-care providers cannot afford to do all these tests on all of their patients. They have to sit with patients and figure out how to lead them to healing. Western medicine is good at trauma, acute infections, replacing joints, and replacing organs, but it is not good for chronic diseases or for helping patients with stress, nutrition, and overall health and well-being.

There was a manual developed in China called *A Barefoot Doctor's Manual.* Peasants were trained to go into the rural areas and practice basic medicine and heal basic illnesses. They were taught preventative medicine by trained doctors who didn't want to go to these rural areas. They were called barefoot doctors because they used to walk barefoot through the fields. A health coach is a modern-day barefoot doctor and an integral part of the future of medicine. Doctors and coaches are partnering to bring the best care to patients and clients that they possibly can. Doctors are slowly realizing that coaches are the missing link in the sustainability of healthful recommendations.

It is rare for anyone to get an hour with a trained professional to work on his or her nutrition and goals. As a health coach, I create a supportive environment that enables clients to achieve all of their health goals. I have studied all the major dietary theories, and I use practical lifestyle coaching methods to guide my clients in discovering which approach works best for them.

Most approaches to nutrition dwell on calories, carbs, fats, and proteins. Instead of creating lists of restrictions and good and bad foods, I coach my clients to create a happy, healthy life in a way that is flexible and fun. My approach is not to take away foods but to add foods. Eventually, the healthy foods crowd out the not-so-healthy stuff.

MY ROLE AS A COACH

As a coach, I guide you to find the food and lifestyle choices that best support *you*. I also help you to make gradual, lifelong changes that enable you to reach your current and future health goals.

We all deserve a life of joy; a healthy mind, body, and spirit; a sense of purpose; and meaningful relationships. Sometimes we become dissatisfied with our lives, and this dissatisfaction can be an indication that something is out of balance. We feel stuck, unsure, or possibly overwhelmed with a new situation. We feel *stressed*. Other times, we are motivated and have new energy to achieve a personal goal, but we don't know what steps to take to get there, and soon our motivation dwindles. This is a very frustrating state.

Health and happiness come from our primary and secondary foods. When one area is off, look at another area, and often you can find a solution. For example, let's say you are having trouble losing weight. Maybe you have a troubling relationship, you hate your job, you don't exercise, and God seems to be in a galaxy far, far away. On top of that, the food you put in your body lacks the nutrients you need for a healthy mind and body. Nourishment comes from all these elements combined. We single them out, somehow thinking they are not connected in any way. It is all connected, all the time.

The coaching adventure begins with creating your vision of your best self through a process involving inquiry and intention. Next, coach and client work together to create a wellness plan that offers direction toward fulfilling your goals through an ongoing relationship with your health coach that includes encouragement, self-evaluation, skill building, practice, and accountability. Much like a runner training for a big race, the wellness plan is comparable to a training schedule individually designed to direct you toward success. Together, coach and client explore ways to maintain balance and ultimately thrive in all areas of wellness, including

- **physical fitness and healthy diet:** exercise, nutrition, sleep, stress management
- **mental and emotional fitness:** self-awareness, positive coping strategies, resilience, social support, spirituality, and navigating life's challenges
- **professional fulfillment:** living your life's passion, contributing your talents and skills, managing time
- **healthy relationships:** communication, boundaries, intimacy, respect
- **values clarification and healthy decision making:** understanding your priorities, keeping your commitments to yourself and others

A health coach assists you in a positive, encouraging, inquisitive manner, so *you* can

- **gain self-awareness**, self-confidence, and strategies for lasting change
- **prioritize your goals** to achieve your vision of success
- **stay focused and in control** of your destiny

I don't help people to NOT die. I help them to enjoy
and love their life.

—BERNIE SIEGAL

ONE SIMPLE CHANGE

Hire a health coach today. Most approaches to healthy eating dwell
on calories, carbohydrates, fats, and proteins. Instead of creating lists
of restrictions and good and bad foods, I coach my clients to explore
basic improvements and implement gradual changes during our work
together. As these changes accumulate, my clients find that the changes
collectively have a much larger impact than they originally expected.
We work on what you want to improve, and we focus on your unique
situation.

Together we will

- connect the dots between who you are and who you want to be,
- create your personal blueprint,
- decipher your body's unique needs,
- set your personal goals and work toward sustainable change,
- identify your personal challenges, and
- reduce your stress in order to push past the obstacles holding
  you back from your best life.

CHAPTER 2

NURTURE YOURSELF WITH MASSAGE

Cast all your anxiety on him because he cares for you.

—1 PETER 5:7 (NIV)

STRESS IS UNIVERSAL, and it's not always bad. Whenever you jump to catch a badly thrown ball, feel especially energetic before an important meeting, or hit the brakes in time to avoid a car accident, stress is doing its job. The adrenaline boosting your heart rate and the cortisol boosting your blood sugar, while diverting energy away from your digestive system and immune responses, are exactly what humans need to either fight or flee.

However, when there's never any relief from stress, the sustained fight-or-flight response can cause problems. Constant stress actually becomes distress—a negative stress reaction. Distress can lead to physical symptoms including headaches, upset stomach, elevated blood pressure, chest pain, and problems sleeping. Research suggests that stress can also bring on or worsen certain symptoms or diseases.

When our bodies are overstressed, they give off what I like to call "enlisting help indicators." Here are three areas to watch for:

Behavior changes
- Angry outbursts
- Drug or alcohol abuse

- Over- or undereating
- Social withdrawal
- Tobacco use

Mood changes
- Anxiety
- Irritability or anger
- Lack of motivation or focus
- Restlessness
- Sadness or depression

Body changes
- Chest pain
- Fatigue
- Headache
- Muscle tension or pain
- Reduced sex drive, low libido
- Difficulty sleeping, falling asleep, or staying asleep all night
- Stomach upset

If you are experiencing these symptoms on any level, it is time to slow down and make the necessary changes to reduce your stress.

MASSAGE THERAPY AND STRESS

Virtually every symptom our bodies experience because of stress can benefit from massage. Research has shown that it can lower your heart rate and blood pressure, relax your muscles, and increase the production of endorphins, your body's natural, feel-good chemical. Serotonin and dopamine are also released through massage, and the result is a feeling of calm relaxation that makes chronic or habitual stress, as well as acute or short-term stress, much easier to overcome.

In fact, stress relief is one of the first benefits that come to mind when thinking of massage therapy. It's also a key component for anyone trying to achieve a healthier lifestyle. Clinical studies show that even a single one-and-a-half-hour session can significantly lower your heart rate, cortisol levels, and insulin levels—all of which explain why massage therapy and stress relief go hand in hand.

BENEFITS OF MASSAGE THERAPY FOR STRESS

Taking care of your body should be at the top of your list of priorities. By adding therapeutic massage to your routine now, you'll feel, look, and simply be healthier far into the future. In fact, stress relief alone can improve your vitality and state of mind. So what better way to prep for a long, happy life than a relaxing, therapeutic massage?

ONE SIMPLE CHANGE

One of the best things I do for myself anytime, but especially during times of high stress, is to get a massage. During these times, I go once a week, but the benefits can be significant even if you can only go once every four to six weeks. If you are going through a stressful time, add massage therapy or increase the frequency of your massage therapy as a way to cope with and counter the harmful effects that stress can have on your mind and body. Massage Envy is one of many membership-based establishments that offer massage at a reduced rate. Most massage schools also offer massage at a significant cost reduction. See it as a necessary, preventative measure. You are worth the investment.

RETREAT OFTEN

Stress can be caused by both good and bad experiences—the damaging effects are the same. When stress comes from unpleasant experiences, tensions, conflicts, or even devastating experiences like the death of a loved one, we think these experiences will kill us. We naturally take steps to avoid them. However, the stress that comes from experiences that are exciting and challenging can also lead to our destruction. These stressors keep us so wired and create such a pleasant experience, we don't think of taking steps to remove the stress. You have probably seen seemingly happy people having the time of their lives, partying all night and sleeping all day or sleeping very little. They say they are having a good time, and it would appear that they are, but inside, their minds and bodies are ticking time bombs ready to go off and cause mental and physical breakdown.

Failure to give our bodies time to push the reset button or failure to recharge our bodies' energy levels after a time of stress is disastrous to our health. If you never give your body time to heal, catch up, and get back to your original state of being, you will find yourself in a state of complete exhaustion. You need rest times; you need a day off; you need to take periodic vacations; and it is vital to build in time for a personal retreat.

ONE SIMPLE CHANGE

One thing I do frequently is a staycation. This is a vacation, but you stay in town where you live. I will often stay at a hotel in downtown Houston, and it feels like I am somewhere else. While you're on staycation, order room service, watch a movie, take a nap, take long strolls in a new park you have never been to, rent a city bike, and explore the town you live in. In fact, you do not even need to book a hotel for a staycation. You can stay at home as long as you are mindful about how you spend your time. Don't worry about errands and cleaning. If you have children, send them to a friend or family member's for a weekend visit. Don't feel guilty about staying in your room to catch up on that book you have been wanting to read or those magazines you never seem to have the time to get to. You get the idea. Whatever you do, relax, rest, and enjoy life.

CHAPTER 3

DRINK UP

So whether you eat or drink or whatever you do, do it all
for the glory of God.

—1 Corinthians 10:31 (NIV)

I HAD PRETTY bad morning sickness when I was pregnant with both of my kids, first with Lily and then with Nathan, who was born December 14, 2005. When I was pregnant with my son, it was more like an all-day, every-day-for-nine-months sickness. For the first five months, the morning sickness was severe. I threw up every day several times a day.

Just as the nausea was beginning to ease up, we took a planned trip to Washington State to visit family. I was tired most of the time and not able to do much of anything except continue to nurture the baby I was carrying inside me.

The day before we were to return home, I went into a heart arrhythmia called atrial fibrillation. I ended up in the hospital for two days. When I got there, I was severely dehydrated, and doctors suspected this was contributing to the arrhythmia. It was astonishing how many fluids they pumped into me intravenously—and it still took two days for my heart to return to a normal rhythm. It was frightening to think that my life and my baby were in jeopardy because I was not well hydrated.

This is just one example of the importance of hydration. Our bodies are made up of about 70 percent water, which is involved in every bodily function.

WATER

Dehydration is not an option for me. If I am not properly hydrated, I get heart palpitations, which leave me feeling tired and anxious and like I have a fish flopping around in my chest. As you can imagine, I am a heavy drinker of water. I carry a flask wherever I go. You could call me an *aquaholic*.

Doctors have told me that my metabolism mows through electrolytes at a faster than average rate. Electrolytes (examples include minerals like potassium and sodium) are ionized or ionizable constituents of cells, blood, or other organic matter. They are key elements of true hydration and need water to be absorbed by our cells. Add a bit of sea salt to your water to mineralize it and add electrolytes. This will help your cells absorb the water better, resulting in full hydration. Coconut water is another great source of electrolytes and a great hydrator. It has been called nature's Gatorade!

Herbal teas are another great way to get hydrated with a little extra boost. I drink green tea in the morning, which gives me that natural caffeine boost plus lots of antioxidants. Later in the day, I go for caffeine-free tea, such as a chamomile or mint. Chamomile can help with stress, and mint provides energy—both are tasty ways to stay hydrated.

I'm lucky to live in an area with safe, good-tasting tap water. If you feel your water is not from a good, clean source or if it doesn't taste good, use a water filter.

It astonished me the first time I learned how much of my physical and mental well-being was linked to how well hydrated I was. Not being properly hydrated makes the blood thicker, increasing the risk for clotting and making it harder to pump it through the system. This can have a serious impact on blood pressure and heart disease. Lack of water is also linked to headaches, joint pain, and muscle tension. It even causes stomachaches, heartburn, stress, anxiety, and depression. All of your systems are connected throughout the body, and it's important not to neglect one of this network's most important tools.

If you suffer from any of the following ailments, you may not be drinking enough water: fatigue, confusion, memory loss, dizziness, dry and wrinkled skin, brittle hair and nails, cold fingers and toes, constipation, eczema, headaches, urinary tract infections, muscle pains, and even anxiety and depression. These are all signs of dehydration. Below are six very good reasons to boost your water intake:

1. You will digest your food better.

If you're spending a bit too much time and effort on the toilet, you could probably use a glass (or two!) of pure water. The body is very wise: it knows that the vital organs need essential nutrients more than the rest of your body.

If you're dehydrated, your body's organs and cells will take what's available. Hence, constipation. Water-depleted stools are hard to pass—and they can be there for days! As a result, your digestive tract feels bloated with an overgrowth of fermenting bacteria and yeast. Not fun!

2. You will stay sharp.

If you prefer being upbeat and focused, you need to drink water. If you're feeling confused and forgetful, try drinking more water before going to see the doctor. Dehydration can trigger brain fog. It makes you feel groggy, hungry, and generally just *off*.

Water is a calming agent for all of our bodily systems; it reduces and minimizes stress. After all, it is necessary for providing our cells with micronutrients vital to biological processes. If those functions are compromised, your body will experience stress. It doesn't take long for your mind to pick up on this physical stress, making it hard to focus. Your brain is trying to tell you to get up and get something to drink.

3. You will love what you see in the mirror.

If you love what you see in the mirror every morning, good for you! Keep doing what you're doing! But if you are met with a puffy face, sunken eyes, or dark, under-eye circles, take it as a warning that your kidneys are in distress. You are not drinking enough water. Without adequate hydration, your body will try to get moisture from any liquid source in your system. It will automatically tap your blood, cell fluid, intracellular fluid, and even your stools and urine. When you've literally drained yourself, you'll be affecting your physical and mental health. This places tremendous stress on the body and mind, and this physical and mental stress speeds up the aging process.

The kidneys filter toxins, salts, and excess water from the bloodstream. If the body is dehydrated, the kidneys can't function properly. If the kidneys are overloaded, your face will reveal it. Maybe you had a fun night out with a bit too much booze. Maybe you ate too many salty snacks, or maybe you've been ingesting too much sodium from takeout food. Whatever the reason, the result is written all over your face.

4. YOU WILL HAVE YOUTHFUL SKIN.

Dry and wrinkled skin occurs for two big reasons: (1) water retention and (2) a lack of subcutaneous fat. If you want to boost your skin's natural fillers, look more youthful, and restore that healthy glow, do three things:

1. Splash cool water on your face several times every morning.
2. Gently pat your skin dry.
3. Drink a big glass of water on an empty stomach.

Make sure you drink more than two liters of water and eat fat every day! By *fat*, I mean pure and unprocessed plant oils from foods like organic flax seeds, butter from grass-fed sources, avocados, and organic coconut oil. Skip the greasy bacon and cookies with partially hydrogenated oils! Fat binds the water to the dermis of the skin, which functions as a natural filler. The fat will be stored in this layer and prevent that hollow look that often appears with age. It's nature's Botox!

5. YOU WILL LOWER YOUR BODY FAT.

This will probably surprise you, but being dehydrated can make you gain weight. As I mentioned earlier, the body will use all other fluids available when it's dehydrated. Water is a natural appetite suppressant, and it regulates your metabolism. When you are dehydrated, your metabolism slows down, affecting how your body burns fat. When you are thirsty, your body is tricked into thinking it is hungry, which then leads to increased calorie consumption. This shows up in an increase in belly fat.

When you are dehydrated, the kidneys become stressed because they cannot filter toxins. The liver then becomes stressed and metabolizes fat more slowly.

Dehydration also messes with your hormones. Testosterone levels decrease, and insulin production increases when you are dehydrated, leading to excessive fat being stored.

6. YOU WILL CURB YOUR APPETITE.

Do you constantly feel hungry? Do you have cravings for sugar and junk food? Drink a glass of water. Pure water acts as an appetite suppressant. When you feel hungry, I suggest you drink a big glass of water before you act on that sensation. If you need some flavor, you can add a bit of lemon juice or a splash of acai or pomegranate juice (without any added sugar).

ONE SIMPLE CHANGE

How much water do you need? In general, you need about two liters (sixty-five ounces) of pure water a day. The best way to ensure you get enough is to plan ahead and check in with yourself throughout the day. To get off to a good start, drink two glasses of water upon rising in the morning and two glasses before consuming each meal of the day. Stop drinking water three to four hours before bedtime, so you won't disrupt your sleep. Be sure to consider other factors that affect how much water your body needs. For example, you might need more if you are in a warm or dry climate or if you exercise often or intensely. Plus, take into account the diuretic effects of coffee, tea, alcohol, and sodas, as well as the dehydrating effect of salty foods. To compensate for these things,

I follow the rule that for every eight ounces of caffeinated beverage or every serving of salty snack, I need eight ounces of water to break even.

CONSIDER CAFFEINE

I often joke that water is the most essential element of life because without it, you cannot make coffee.

I love coffee. I love the smell of it, the taste of it, and the whole ritual of preparing it. I love the pleasure of drinking it with friends, all by myself in a coffee shop, or on the porch of a fine hotel. I just plain love coffee. I call it my happy juice. Drinking coffee or other caffeinated beverages can create a sense of increased energy, sharper focus, and a happier mood—effects that will last for a couple of hours. But after that, it wears off, and you're left with an aftermath of anxiety, low energy, and a depressed mood. I learned that caffeine is a stimulant and a huge trigger for anxiety. Plus, it is a diuretic that pulls water out of our cells. I had to find a solution so that I could still indulge in coffee but not feed the caffeine beast, which triggers my anxiety and stress. If you experience a lot of stress in your life, caffeine will inevitably create anxiety, and you should consider eliminating coffee or reducing your intake of it. I am very sensitive to caffeine and had to accept that it was not something I could drink every day—and certainly not in large amounts—because it amplified my anxiety immensely.

ONE SIMPLE CHANGE

My solution to reducing my caffeine intake was to switch to coffee that is decaffeinated through a natural, water-based process. (My favorite is Café Altura's organic decaf.) I also increased my intake of naturally caffeinated herbal teas, such as yerba mate and green tea, which contain far less caffeine than regular coffee. I also drink a lot of naturally decaffeinated herbal teas, such as chamomile. This mix and a few simple swaps have worked for me. Once in a while, I indulge in the *real thing* but prepare myself for the fact that I may experience some anxiety as a result.

CHAPTER 4

BREATHE DEEPLY

The spirit of God has made me; the breath of the
Almighty gives me life.

—Job 33:4 (NIV)

Adopt the pace of nature; her secret is patience.

—Ralph Waldo Emerson

ONE OF THE best things my mother taught me was to breathe deeply to relieve stress and anxiety. Let me tell you, it works. Deep breathing is one of the best and most natural tranquilizers there is. It is nearly impossible for stress to remain present when you are practicing deep breathing. You may have noticed that if you are in a stressful situation, perhaps when someone is annoying you, you take a deep breath and blow it out forcefully. Even though you are feeling exasperated, the deep breath and the forceful exhalation are your body's attempts to calm itself down. So the next time you have to "huff" at someone, just explain that you are attempting the stress-relieving practice of deep breathing instead of punching him or her in the face. Then, invite him or her to join in. Before you know it, you will be happy, calm, well-oxygenated BFFs.

Breathing resets your emotional state. It's that simple.

Andrew Weil is an American physician, author, and spokesperson, generally described as a holistic health and integrative medicine guru. He talks about the importance of deep breathing in a lecture for IIN. According to Weil, the theory of breath work is that it is the only thing we can do completely consciously or completely unconsciously. It offers us a chance to influence the involuntary nervous system. The theory states that with imposing rhythms on your breath with your voluntary system, you gradually induce those rhythms in the involuntary system, which controls everything. It controls circulation, digestion, and all the functions of the body.

Whether it's for five minutes, fifteen minutes, thirty minutes, or more, it would be ideal to make deep breathing a part of your daily life. You can put this into practice while sitting in traffic, sitting at your desk, or before you fall asleep at night. If you wake up in the middle of the night, it can be a tool you use to help you fall asleep again. Deep breathing can be done anywhere and anytime you feel the need to calm yourself down. You may feel lightheaded at first, but that feeling will disappear with practice. The more important effect you may notice is a sense of relaxation.

If you stick with your breathing regimen and practice it consistently, if not every day, without fail, I promise you that in six to eight weeks, you will begin to see changes that are quite remarkable. Studies have shown that after incorporating deep breathing, people who used to have cold hands all the time have warm hands. High blood pressure normalizes, and chronic digestion disorders are reduced or disappear as a direct result of deliberate deep breathing. It is the most powerful antianxiety measure I have ever found.

Let me say that I think there is a time and place for medication. I know that change can be a huge trigger for stress, anxiety, and depression. Moving, a job loss or change, the death of a loved one, illness, divorce, and other major life events can bring on unexpected responses in our physical and mental well-being. Sometimes we need a little extra help. Even if a person is doing everything right, she might still struggle in the face of enormous pressures that are beyond her control. It is possible to be so far down that it takes extra help to bring us to a place where we feel we can even make the move toward adopting healthy coping mechanisms. Modern medicine has given us some wonderful options to pair with more natural forms of stress, anxiety, and depression management.

You do not have to suffer, thinking you should manage such immense changes on your own. When clients come to me for health coaching, I often team up with their doctors to develop a wellness plan. Together, we can get them on the road to their best life. I am currently on an antianxiety medication that I started taking after my mom died. At the time, I felt as if I was going to die. I ended up in the ER three times due to anxiety; I thought I was having a heart attack. Making decisions became agonizing because I was fearful of making the wrong one. I was doing all the right things—not perfectly—but doing them. The blow of unexpectedly losing my mom knocked me off my feet, and I needed help getting up. Her death triggered major anxiety in me. I describe it as swinging a heavy anchor above my head, around and around. I needed to drop it somewhere, but my ocean was too deep and too wide. My sorrow was heavy and paralyzing. I became depleted and exhausted. Today I am very mindful, each day, of the choices I need to make. Not just to survive and keep the darkness at bay, but to restore calm and experience peace and joy every day.

Try experimenting with deep breathing and the technique I describe in the coming pages. If someone cuts you off in traffic, if someone says something to push your buttons, do the deep-breathing technique before you react. Your reaction is less likely to be volatile. Be patient, and put it into practice daily.

Deep breathing is also a great way to deal with cravings. Practice deep breathing before acting on a craving and then wait twenty minutes. Your craving may disappear or become manageable. The deep breathing changes the tone of your autonomic nervous system in a way that is very desirable, and that is one of the most important effects of deep breathing.

THE DEEP-BREATHING TECHNIQUE

In *The Anxiety Cure,* Hart mentions a deep-breathing technique I have integrated into my own life: Breathe steady and rhythmically for a few minutes. Make sure you are breathing from your abdomen and not your chest. Our breathing shows our stress, and someone who is stressed or anxious will breathe from the upper lungs and chest; his or her breathing will be shallow and rapid. If you are in a relaxed state, you will breathe more deeply and slowly, more from your lower lungs and abdomen. A way to test how you are breathing is to lie down on your back and place your hand on your abdomen just below the ribs. If your hand moves up with your breathing, then you are breathing deeply from your abdomen. If your hand doesn't rise and fall with each breath, then you are chest breathing.

Try not to breathe just from your chest muscles. This is nervous breathing and is designed for a fight-or-flight response in an emergency. It's not sustainable. Try breathing in through your nose and out through your mouth. Proper deep breathing activates the calming, relaxation response in the body. It gives us the ability to change the chemistry of our bodies. This type of breathing allows the air to pass through the turbinates in the nose, aiming the breath at the lower lobes of the lungs. That's where the vagus nerve comes through the diaphragm. When you take a deep breath through the nose, you are automatically firing off the rest-and-restore nervous system.

Calm is a superpower.

When you breathe in, take in as much breath as you can, taking your time. When you breathe out, let as much air out of your lungs as possible, again taking your time. After a few times, breathe normally, and be aware of how your breathing has changed.

When you slow down and pay attention to how you are breathing, you are developing one of the most powerful tools to combat any stressful, anxious situation or state of being. Frequently ask yourself, "How fast am I breathing? Is my breathing shallow or deep? Am I breathing from my chest or abdomen?"

Our very lives may depend on whether we learn how to relax or not. Do not be discouraged if you are not able to do it at first. Keep practicing, and it will eventually come to you. I always tell my children when they are learning something new and feel that they will never get it, "It is hard until you learn it. Once you learn it, it becomes easy."

ONE SIMPLE CHANGE

Set aside time each day for deep breathing. Some people prefer to begin their day with a few minutes of deliberate breathing and relaxation. Others like to use the practice to unwind at bedtime. Be consistent, and practice the technique described in this chapter. At first, you might find you need to make corrections to ensure you are breathing from your abdomen, but with time and practice, it will come naturally. Here are a few tips to keep in mind:

- **Close your eyes.** It is much easier to focus on how your body feels when you are not distracted by the sights around you.
- **Follow your breath.** As you inhale, feel the air as it enters your nose and travels deep into your lower lungs. As you exhale, feel your breath moving up through your chest and out of your body.
- **Work from top to bottom.** Once you begin to feel relaxed, check in with each part of your body to release any stress you are holding there. Begin with your head, paying special attention to your forehead, jaw, and the back of your head just above your neck. Then, move down to your neck and shoulders; then, move down your arms to your fingertips. Move to your core, focusing on your back, spine, and hips, before working your way down your legs to your feet and toes.

You can sneak a short deep-breathing session into the middle of your day. This is especially helpful if you are feeling stressed. With time, you will become attuned to your body and become more aware of what brings on tension.

CHAPTER 5

ADOPT A MEDITATION PRACTICE

May the words of my mouth and this meditation of my
heart be pleasing in your sight, Lord, my Rock and my
Redeemer.

—Psalm 19:14 (NIV)

Regular meditation has the ability to cause the brain to
re-orient itself from a stressful fight-or-flight mode to
one of acceptance, a shift that increases contentment.
You don't need a guru to find the secret of centered-
ness. All you have to do is breathe.

—Maia Szalavitz

I remember one of the first times I took a yoga class. At the end of the
class, there was a time of meditation. The instructor told us to pick a
position that was comfortable for us, and I chose to be flat on my back.
She guided us through a progressive relaxation technique that kept us
in the present moment. The exercise lasted only a few minutes, but I was
so relaxed that I kept falling asleep. I would wake up briefly, still in a
state of extreme relaxation, and then drift off again. That happened five
times! I had these micro dreams, one about Adrien Brody (an actor),

one about making kale salad, and one about sex that luckily involved neither Brody nor kale. How's that for meditation?

Meditation has changed and evolved over the years. It's not for weirdos on the fringes, and it's no longer just a religious practice. It is simply a wonderful way to stop, breathe, notice, reflect, and respond. It can most definitely be a time of connection to our Creator, and I strongly encourage this. After all, our bodies, according to the Bible, are temples for the Holy Spirit to dwell in us. What better way to engage in that wonderful relationship than to stop, slow down, and take time to meditate?

Getting people to relax is one of the objectives of meditation. The other objective is to get people to focus their awareness on the present moment. This can be difficult to do when you are first learning to meditate, but over time you learn how to calm your mind and body and still be fully present. When this happens, it's a wonderful feeling. It's like being super alive, like when you're really enjoying something or totally focused on the task.

My usual waking state is just the opposite. I tend to have a "monkey mind" (a Buddhist term for an unsettled, restless, inconstant, confused, indecisive, or uncontrolled mind), or I tend to daydream, so I'm rarely completely present in the moment. I'm either worrying about what I need to do next or I'm totally checked out.

It's OK if this happens to you, but if you practice meditation consistently enough, you are bound to experience moments when you are present in the moment. Meditation can put you in a state of mindfulness, strengthen your ability to resolve conflict, and make you more restfully available to love more, love deeper, and love better. [2]Tim Ryan, author of *A Mindful Nation*, says, "If more citizens can reduce stress and increase performance, they will be better equipped to face the challenges of daily life and to arrive at creative solutions to the challenges facing our nation." He claims it is a matter of national security.

Back in the 1970s, best-selling author Herbert Benson argued in *The Relaxation Response* that people who meditated could counteract the

---

2 Joel Stein, "Just say Om," *Time: Your body*, Collectors Edition (November 22, 2013): 24

stress-induced fight-or-flight response and achieve a calmer, happier state. Simply by focusing on the present moment, people who meditate can control the way their brains receive input.

All people who meditate may experience the same benefits, but as with many aspect of wellness, meditation is driven by bio-individuality, which means that what works for each person is unique. There isn't any one true way to receive its benefits.

I have found that, as with exercise or diet, the right routine is the one that you will make a regular part of your life. Meditation can be as simple as inhaling and exhaling. It can be done when walking or running or doing any type of rhythmic or repetitive activity. Listening to calming music, such as classical, jazz, or Spanish guitar music, can evoke a mindful, meditative state. As for me, when I first started meditating, I put a lot of pressure on myself to feel a certain way. I thought that if I meditated, I would experience a special something, and if I didn't, I must be doing it wrong. This is a very common feeling, but it is incorrect. The whole point of meditating is to simply notice the play of the mind and body and not get bent out of shape when things are not perfect. I recommend trying to meditate for about five to fifteen minutes to start. That's just enough time to get really bored. Learn how to make room for unpleasant moments.

Meditation isn't about achieving some goal or doing something correctly so that you can perform better in another part of your life. Mindful meditation is not about getting somewhere now. It is about being where you are and knowing it. So much of our behavior is motivated by urges going on below the surface of our awareness. It's as if we're saying to ourselves, "Give me more" or "Get me out of here." But if we can learn to be mindful, those forces become far less stressful, and both our physical and mental health can improve, no matter what our circumstances. I do believe the Bible calls this joy. Joy is not the same as happiness.

Everything we do is infused with the energy with which we do it. If we are frantic, life will be frantic. If we are peaceful, life will be peaceful.

You can start meditating anywhere, anytime, just by focusing on your breathing. Of course, the best time to begin is now.

Here is one of my go-to meditations. At any point in your day, stop and do a body tension inventory. What I mean by that is to sit and quiet your mind, close your eyes, and take a deep breath. Start from your head, and work your way down to your toes. Ask yourself along your body journey, "Where am I holding tension?" Then release the tension through breath. This can be a five-minute exercise or take longer if you really need to decompress. It is a game changer.

Sonia Chochette, a meditation teacher with more than thirty-five years of experience, says, [3]"When you meditate, you put your guard down, let energy in, and get yourself out of a stressful self-defense mode. Meditation is pressing a pause button and giving yourself room to breathe. And when you have room to breathe, you access your greater potential and your greater state of being."

Gabrielle Berstein, a certified meditation teacher and *New York Times* best-selling author, says, [4]"It can also even out your mood and energy levels." Bernstein notes that when we meditate, "We experience more even-keeled energy…And that expands to how we show up in the world. Plus, it may even help you save money on your health care."

Here are nine proven benefits of meditation:

1. ALLEVIATE DEPRESSION

Research suggests that thirty minutes of meditation improves depression symptoms (along with anxiety and pain). In fact, the practice could possibly prevent depression and pain altogether. In a scientific study in 2013 at Brown University, scientists discovered that people who meditate may have more control over how their brains process and pay attention to negative sensations (like pain) and negative thoughts (like depression triggers).

---

3 "19 Science-backed reasons to meditate," Alexandra Duron, The Greatist, December 31, 2014, http://greatist.com/grow/science-backed-reasons-meditate

4 "19 Science-backed reasons to meditate," Alexandra Duron, The Greatist, December 31, 2014, http://greatist.com/grow/science-backed-reasons-meditate

2. DE-STRESS

Nix those nail-biting moments. When you meditate, you're able to override a part of the brain responsible for the fear mechanism, which releases cortisol, the damaging stress hormone that's responsible for a whole grab bag of health issues. One study at Wake Forest Medical Center suggests that meditation can reduce anxiety by almost 40 percent. And it doesn't take a ton of time to reap these keep-calm-and-carry-on benefits. Just twenty-five minutes of meditation done three times per week may make tasks feel less stressful.

3. IMPROVE YOUR MEMORY

If your desktop is wallpapered with sticky note reminders and you often find your mind jumping from thought to thought, you may want to turn to meditation. It's been shown to not only improve memory but also help cut back on distracting thoughts.

4. MAXIMIZE YOUR WORKOUT

Ben Turshen, a former lawyer who's now a fitness professional and qualified independent teacher of Vedic meditation in New York City, says that exercise, especially high-intensity interval (HIIT) training workouts in full-blown beast mode, can do a number on your muscles and your central nervous system, but meditation allows you to rest your body and mind very deeply, removing stress from your system and priming you for excellent sweat sessions. Because of meditation's ability to reduce our stress levels, we're able to perform our workouts that much better and enjoy them that much more, he says.

5. BUILD BETTER BONDS

Meditation will help you maintain healthy relationships. It not only lets you be more present in relationships but also helps you approach tricky situations with a calm mind and body. In fact, it may help you avoid big blowouts when dealing with a relationship issue. One study in 2012 at the University of California, San Francisco, showed people who meditated and tried to problem solve with their partners approached the issue with less hostility and a better mood.

6. SHIELD YOUR HEART

Here's a pretty great (and totally unexpected) way to boost your heart health. That's right, meditation. In one study, patients with coronary heart disease who practiced meditation had a reduced risk of heart attack, stroke, and even depression.

7. GET MORE SLEEP

In a world where we take our phones and tablets to bed, shut-eye has become a pretty precious thing. The problem? Quieting the mind enough to actually be able to fall asleep. That's where meditation comes in. Not only does science suggest it may help treat insomnia, experts also believe that meditating can help keep your mind in check throughout the day and reduce stress, thus leading to a better, more restful night's sleep.

8. BOOST CREATIVITY AND PRODUCTIVITY

The possible cure for a creative rut? Meditation. When you're in a listening state of mind, you put yourself in a position to receive new ideas and inspiration that you weren't able to receive before because you were guarded and protected. So new ideas, solutions, and "aha!" moments will start pouring in. And science agrees: In April 2012, a study at Leiden University, "Meditate to Create: The Impact of Focused-Attention and Open-Monitoring Training on Convergent and Divergent Thinking," found that participants who practiced a particular kind of meditation were better at coming up with many possible solutions for a problem. Meditation has also been shown to help office workers multi-task, remember what tasks they need to complete, and keep their stress levels low.

9. GET THAT YOUTHFUL GLOW

The fountain of youth is as real as calorie-free cookies (imagine a sad-faced emoji here), but meditating may actually help make you younger. Middle-aged participants who practiced meditation had younger biological ages than those who didn't. A fascinating study was conducted by scientist Elizabeth Blackburn. In 2009 she won the Nobel Prize for her discovery of the protective caps on chromosomes, called "telomeres." Every time a cell divides, these protective caps wear down, and over time, the telomeres shorten. As the telomeres shorten, the cells start to malfunction and lose their ability to divide. One of the biggest contributors to the shortening of telomeres is...you guessed it. Stress. Today, based on Blackburn's research, scientists use the measure of telomere length as a metric for aging and disease risk. Blackburn conducted a study on the effects of meditation on telomere length. The results were impressive. There was a significant lengthening of telomeres in those who had a regular practice of meditation.

My meditation practice takes on many forms. Sometimes I just sit in a quiet place and focus on my breathing or on a Bible scripture. I may repeat or focus on a word such as *calm* or *peace* or *relax*. I sometimes take a walk in nature and just meditate and appreciate the sights, sounds, and smells of my surroundings. I often include prayer and yoga with my meditation. Find what works you. It you are thinking that meditation is for new age, goo goo, la la, crazy, chanting people, think again. It is not. It is a time-out period when you refocus, relax, and recharge your brain for your epic life.

ONE SIMPLE CHANGE

I recommend starting with five minutes of meditation—no more and no less—for one week. Five minutes is an easy win, which always feels awesome. Get used to the idea of meditating. Be mindful of how you feel and of the thoughts and sensations, uncomfortable or otherwise, you experience. If you do more than the recommended time and have a negative experience or feel uncomfortable, you may be less motivated to do it consistently or at all. Setting a realistic, attainable goal of five minutes is a good place to start. Set a timer, preferably one that is silent, since hearing the seconds ticking away can really take you out of the moment. Don't forget to breathe.

CHAPTER 6

SLEEP WELL

In peace I will lie down and sleep, for you alone, Lord,
make me dwell in safety.

—Psalm 4:8 (NIV)

A good laugh and a long sleep are the best cures for just
about anything.

—Wendy Lee Jaques

Raising children from birth to about age three is what I call the boot-camp phase. One of the most notable stressors during this time is lack of sleep. There were moments during this phase when I would look at my husband and feel completely repulsed. I loved my children, but I felt that all this feeding, pooping, and lack of sleep were highly inconvenient. I loved them, but I did not like them. I knew this phase would pass, but I was so tired and drained that I wanted to break up with my husband and send the baby to boarding school. It was not the best time ever!

If I do not get enough good-quality sleep, the whole color of my world changes. Bright, peaceful, double rainbows become the black swirling center of a tornado. If you get close enough to me when I am in this state of being, you'll wish that you had never even met me. If I ever find myself in this place, it is all hands on deck, requiring a major *intervention*. If you love me enough, you will gather the family and announce that "the girl needs some sleep, or someone is going to die!" (My intervention would preferably include a two-week stint in Arizona at Miraval Resort and Spa. I would go peaceably.) But seriously, you have to have a plan and be intentional about taking time for yourself, or the boot-camp phase (and any other stressful phase) has the potential to be a not very fun time.

When I was sick, sleep was critical to my healing. When we sleep, our bodies literally heal themselves.

PREPARE FOR SLEEP

It has been my experience that my evening preparation has a direct effect on the quality of my sleep. From the bed and sheets I sleep on to how long I brush my teeth, several things increase the likelihood that I will have a good night's sleep. These are my top ten sleep hygiene tips:

1. Make sure you have a good, comfortable bed. This is one of the best investments you will make. Buy it new, never used.
2. Make sure you have good-quality, comfortable sheets. I discovered that Wamsutta's 100 percent Supima cotton 725-thread count or higher are the most luxurious for me.
3. Do your nightly hygiene in private. Have it be a time of self-nurturing and quiet retreat.
4. Dim the lights, and eliminate any sources of artificial light such as the television, the computer screen, or a brightly lit alarm clock. This is the time for calm and decompression, not stimulation. Make your room as dark as possible. Even a little light can disrupt your sleep.
5. Avoid stimulants such as sugar and caffeine several hours before bed. Avoid drinking lots of water too close to bedtime so that you are not up for potty breaks all night.
6. Try to keep the same bedtime every night. Your body has a certain rhythm, and it operates best under that rhythm.

7. Give your body time to digest your meal, and avoid eating at least two to three hours before bedtime. Sleep is a time for repair; it is a time when your body rests after working all day. Everything slows down, including digestion. You do not want to have food in your system because it will end up putrefying in your tummy. Yuck! Sometimes, if I am under a lot of stress or coming down with something, I will just eat a light snack instead of dinner a couple of times a week to give my body extra time to rest.

8. Dim the lights at least thirty minutes before bedtime. This triggers the calming, sleepy chemicals in your brain, such as melatonin.

9. Take a hot bath or a hot shower with some calming scents such as chamomile, lavender, or another scent that you like. Light a candle as you soak.

10. Your bedroom should be a sanctuary—a place you enter to rest. Make it a place you love to go to. After all, you spend a good portion of your life there. Keep it clean and free of dust. Keep it nicely decorated, well organized, and free of clutter.

ONE SIMPLE CHANGE

How much you sleep and the quality of your sleep will affect nearly every aspect of your life, so it is vital to get the sleep you need every night. Good sleep is critical to stress management, overall health, and well-being. Practice my suggested sleep hygiene habits consistently, and see how they make you feel after even just one night. Tweak them, experiment, and create your own sleep hygiene ritual.

CHAPTER 7

LOVE MORE

Do not seek revenge or bear a grudge against anyone among your people, but love your neighbor as yourself.

—Leviticus 19:18 (NIV)

The primary agenda of human beings is connection and retaining connection. Stress in our relationships creates anxiety. Anxiety is triggered by a ruptured connection. When we are not connected we are scared and we get defensive. We are always trying to regain that original connection, restore it and retain it.

—Edward Tronick

Edward Tronick, a child psychologist and director of the Child Development Unit at Harvard University, performed an experiment in which he had a mother and her young child interact with each other. In the experiment, the mother would play with the child, who was happy and engaged. Then Tronick had the mother look away, stare in another direction, and not interact with the child. The child tried to get the mother's attention by smiling, laughing, and reaching for the mother. Eventually, the child became distressed and fussy, trying everything to get the mother to engage. Then the mother looked at the child but just stared at the child without engaging. The child became even more distressed and confused about why the mother was not engaging with him, and his demeanor changed, reflecting his stress. As soon as the mother returned to smiling and playing with the child, the child almost immediately returned to his happy, cooing self. Even at a young age, our nature is to have human connection. As Sue Johnson, author of *Love Sense*, says, [5]"We are born very vulnerable needing care, we need to feel valued by other people, and we need to know that we matter. If we call and no one comes, we die."

All of us want a sense of connectedness. We want to feel connected to ourselves; to our spouses; and to our children, friends, and family. One of our greatest human needs is to feel a connection with the ones we love. This includes our friendships and a support system in our community. Our purpose and value as human beings rides on the sense of feeling this connection with others. Connecting is our deepest desire, and losing that connection it is our greatest fear.

THERE IS A NURTURING POWER IN CONNECTION

Regaining lost connections requires safety, for without safety, we are anxious, and when we are anxious, we are defensive, and when we are defensive, we will interrupt our attempts to reestablish a relationship. This causes the cycle to repeat; the new broken connection sends us back to the starting point where a ruptured connection created the anxiety to begin with.

Whether positive or negative, what you affirm grows. What you pay attention to becomes larger. The opposite is true as well. What you focus on in another person can release either the feel-good hormones (endorphins) or the stress hormone (cortisol). You can choose what you pay attention to. You can choose to criticize, shame, and blame or you can edify, encourage, and praise and in that way create safety in your conversations, laying the foundation for secure relationships. The put-down is

---

5 "How to make love last in the age of instant gratification," Sue Johnson, mindbodygreen, July 13, 2014, http://www.mindbodygreen.com/search?q=Sue+johnson+on+relationships

toxic to the human ecosystem, including to the person who launches it. As Bernie Siegel says, "If you want to be happy in your life, find a way to make other people happy."

Although romantic connections follow the same cycle, other special rules apply. Sometimes love seems like some sort of strange, partly psychotic mix of sex and sentiment that nobody can understand. When you're in the muddy waters that sometimes come with love, it can seem very complicated. But really it's quite simple. For most of us, the single most motivating force in life is forming connections. That's why arguing with a partner is such a strong, negative experience. It's about more than winning a power struggle or trying to out-rage the other person. Those negative feelings are about some sort of pain, the loss of connection, and the desire to get that connection back. When we feel that a safe, emotional connection has been damaged, our brains go to a place of fear—we fear abandonment and rejection. All of a sudden, we have tunnel vision that tells us our partner is the enemy. The pain of rejection from a person we depend on registers in our brains in the same place and in the same way as physical pain. Stepping on a nail and hearing criticism from a loved one register the same pain in the human brain, and both are danger cues. Successful couples understand that they are scaring each other when they fight. To avoid having an argument spiral out of control, they slow down and tune in to the expressions on their faces, and they start to try to calm and soothe each other.

[6]Sue Johnson, author of *Love Sense,* says, "sex is very important in marriage because it's a bonding behavior. However, sex without emotional connection is like dancing without music."

ONE SIMPLE CHANGE

Love suffers long and is kind; love does not envy; love
does not parade itself, is not puffed up; does not behave
rudely, does not seek its own, is not provoked, thinks

---

6 "How to make love last in the age of instant gratification," Sue Johnson, mindbodygreen, July 13, 2014, http://www.mindbodygreen.com/search?q=Sue+johnson+on+relationships

no evil; does not rejoice in iniquity, but rejoices in the
truth; bears all things, believes all things, hopes all
things, endures all things. Love never fails.

—1 Corinthians 13: 4–8 (NKJV)

Even if most of us do not seem to want to be loved like this, the truth
is that we are all dying for it. Love this way for one week. Be mindful of
this kind of love. Exaggerate and go overboard, and see what happens.
When you feel true love as described here, you can never love too much.

Though I speak with the tongues of men and of angels,
but have not love, I've become sounding brass or a
clanging symbol. And though I have the gift of proph-
ecy, and understand all mysteries and all knowledge,
and though I have all faith, so that I could remove
mountains, but have not love, I am nothing. And
though I bestow all my goods to feed the poor, and
though I give my body to be burned, but have not love,
it profits me nothing."

—1 Corinthians 13:1–3 (NKJV)

Go love strangers, acquaintances, close friends, and family alike. Express
your feelings to them directly and through your actions. When the week
is over, consider how different you feel. Your heart will probably feel full,
giving you a new source of energy and joy. If you feel ready to deepen
your experience, try loving someone you don't think deserves to be
loved. Put your judgment aside and find acceptance, then move past
that to love the person on your own terms.

CHAPTER 8

GET ORGANIZED

For God is not a God of confusion, but of peace.

—1 Corinthians 14:33 (ESV)

Your external environment is a three-dimensional view of what's going on internally for you.

A room holds energy. Our stuff creates energy. The energy in your room, home, or office can support you, making you feel uplifted, creative, successful, and at peace. Alternatively, it can create just the opposite effect, depleting you of energy and health, leaving you feeling overwhelmed, discouraged, depressed, paralyzed, and stressed out!

Clutter and chaos are just symptoms and a reflection of the mental clutter and discomfort you may be experiencing in your body. Clutter in your environment zaps any positive energy out of a room and contributes to a negative energy flow. This is a huge contributor to health issues, financial woes, relationship stress, and even weight gain. Does that sound like a stretch? Think for a moment about how it feels to be surrounded by clutter. It is difficult to find things, hard to keep track of what bills have been paid, and stressful to have unexpected company. Too much stuff is mentally taxing.

Why we create clutter is directly related to what our minds are thinking, how stressed we are, and how we choose to live. This is where, as a professional organizer, I can help. In order to clear up environmental clutter or chaos, you need to gain clarity on internal issues and goals, connect positively with your environment, and change any habits that don't support your goals. Many people find themselves using clutter as a substitute for something important. Whether that something important is an unfulfilled goal or an absent relationship, clutter won't solve the problem. In fact, it will present a whole bunch of new problems. For lasting, positive change, the work must happen from the inside out, starting with your mind, reconnecting with your body, and aligning your environment.

There really is no way around this. *It's all connected, all the time: the mind, the body, the spirit, and the space.* The environments we create are synergistic with our health and with our destruction. The good news is that you have total control when it comes to putting all this back into balance and alignment.

Here are my top four tips on organizing your life:

1. **Simplify your finances:** Keep your finances organized, and stay on a budget. One of the worst feelings is not having a clue about how much you are spending and what you are spending your money on. Use an online budgeting system such as mint.com. It keeps track of all of your expenses, creating accountability and freedom. It is very easy to set up, and it takes very little time to manage.

2. **Set a timer for everything:** Time management is the act or process of planning and exercising conscious control over the amount of time spent on specific activities, and the goal of time management is to increase effectiveness, efficiency, and productivity. I use the timer on my phone for everything. I also block out time on my calendar for everything I need and want to get done for the day. For example, I will schedule time to write for two hours each day. Setting my timer allows me to be fully present in my writing, and my timer can keep track of when it is time to stop. I will set my timer for thirty minutes and do a quick cleanup of one room. Once the thirty minutes is up, I move

to the next room and set my timer again. A friend and I meet weekly for breakfast, but we usually only have an hour to visit. I will set my timer for forty-five minutes so that when it goes off, we know we have fifteen minutes to transition, end our conversation, and say good-bye. It also allows me to be fully present in my time with my friend, honoring her and our time together instead of constantly checking my phone and interrupting the flow of our conversation.

3. **Declutter your kitchen:** In my kitchen I have organizing systems set up in the pantry and cupboards. I make sure I can see everything in my pantry, and I label everything for ease and access. Throw out old, outdated food, and organize the rest in labeled baskets or canisters. Hooks, stackers, baskets, bins, and shelves will allow you to give everything a home. You will know exactly where everything goes. Get rid of excess kitchenware. Do you need two potato peelers and seven spatulas? Do you really need all that Tupperware? A lot of energy can be wasted looking for things or digging through an excessive number of kitchen gadgets.

4. **Get rid of tolerances:** Tolerances come from all areas of life: home/office; relationships/family; car/appliances/equipment; personal finances/income level; work/clients/customers; and body/appearance. Tolerances are people, events, or situations that we put up with even though doing so drains us of energy. Tolerances keep us from living life to our fullest potential. We have a cup of success, but the holes created by our tolerances keep draining our potential. We fill it up, but it just keeps draining out. Tolerances sap our joy and stifle our creativity. For example, if I have a messy car, every time I get into my car, I spend my energy thinking about the dirt instead of about something more creative and positive. If I have a friend who is chronically tardy, I spend a lot of energy on negative feelings and reactions.

What are your tolerances? I am certain you could come up with at least ten, but you probably have one hundred or more. Make a list in each category, and then get to work on getting them out of your life. Free up energy you didn't even know you had, and watch your creativity soar. Here is how you do it:

1. Set a timer for one hour and aim for getting twenty tolerances off your list.
2. Organize your tolerances according to how much time they take. List all that will take fifteen minutes or less. List the ones that will take thirty minutes to an hour. You get the idea. If you have fifteen minutes, pick something from your list and get rid of it.
3. Have a day when all you do is eliminate tolerances.
4. Hire a health coach to help you in your efforts.

Reducing tolerances will free up and repurpose your energy and time so that you can focus on the people and activities that really matter to you.

ONE SIMPLE CHANGE

Get rid of unnecessary stuff, and organize what is left over. Make this a monthly event, focusing on a few different rooms or spaces each time. Once you organize the things you are keeping, give every item a definite place to call home. Put things away as you are finished with them, and spend fifteen minutes at the end of the day putting any stray items back in their places. Make it a habit so that you never reach a point when clutter overwhelms you. You will find that your decluttered space frees up your energy. Instead of coping with the stress of your surroundings, you will have more energy to direct toward the people you love.

CHAPTER 9

SEIZE THE MOMENT

Therefore do not be anxious, saying, "What shall we eat?" or "What shall we drink?" or "What shall we wear?" For the Gentiles seek after all these things, and your heavenly Father knows that you need them all. But seek first the kingdom of God and his righteousness, and all these things will be added to you. Therefore do not be anxious about tomorrow, for tomorrow will be anxious for itself. Sufficient for the day is its own trouble.

—Mathew 6: 31–34 (ESV)

Life is not a dress rehearsal. Life is now. How we live our days is how we live our lives. So get busy living or get busy dying.

—Anonymous

Often we get so busy with life, we forget who we are, what motivates us, and what inspires us. We forget about the things in our lives that release stress and energize us at the same time. Instead, we are so focused on just doing the next thing on our to-do list, we forget to invest in the things that really matter to us. Often we live in the past, stressing about events and pondering things we have no control over. We are so caught up inside our heads, we forget to slow down and live in the moment.

Inhale deeply, and feel your breath fill your lungs. Feel the breeze across your face and through your hair. Identify the aromas that drift through the air. Notice the sights and sounds around you. Observe the different colors you see. Listen for loud sounds and soft sounds. Slow your gait if you're walking, breathe deeply, and take your time. Allow yourself to relish the moment, and do not let anyone or anything steal your joy. We must create moments of true pleasure when we indulge in the here and now and retreat from the there and then.

Here are three ways to release stress and restore energy at the same time:

HAVE FUN

Here is Sheryl Paul's definition of fun: "Any interaction that results in a belly laugh, an orgasm, or both." Seriously! When was the last time you had some high-energy fun? When was the last time you laughed until your tummy hurt and you just completely enjoyed yourself?

Stress comes from being overworked, overlooked, moving, losing your job, coping with the death of a loved one, and suffering through illness. Stress can also come from the thrilling, exciting, fun things in life if they are not tempered with downtime to rest and relax your mind, body, and spirit. However, I think most of us don't have enough fun. Weave some fun into your day, either every day or every week.

Go online and search for fun things to do in your area. Remember what you liked to do for fun when you were a kid, and start there.

DANCE TO INSPIRING MUSIC

Music can heal you, music can make you happy, music touches where a doctor can never go—to the soul.

—JUDY MOWATT, *ROCKSTEADY: THE ROOTS OF REGGAE*

I am happy to report that my inner child is still ageless.

—James Broughton

A wonderful tradition in our family is to have what we call family dance night. We turn on loud dance music and let ourselves go. Some of us look like Ren, and others look more like Willard from the movie *Footloose*, but we get the job of having fun done! Turn on your favorite music, and dance like nobody's watching!

Here is a short list of some of my playlist favorites:

- "Watch Me" (Whip/Nae Nae) by Silento
- "U Can't Touch This" by MC Hammer
- "Shut Up and Dance" by Walk the Moon
- "Celebration" by Kool and the Gang
- "Lean On" by Major Lazor & DJ Snake
- "Crazy in Love" by Sophia Kalberg
- "Uptown Funk" by Mark Ronson
- "Word Up" by Cameo
- "Pump Up the Jam" by Technotronic
- "What Is Love?" by Haddaway
- "Hold My Hand" by Jess Glynne
- "Party in the USA" by Miley Cyrus
- Any song by Michael Jackson
- Just about anything country

UNPLUG EVERY DAY

When I was sick, I was hypersensitive to almost everything: light, sounds, smells, tastes, and everything I touched. All my senses were on overload. It did get better, but I have developed a great need to keep things calm, quiet, and simple. I allow myself time each day to check e-mails, engage in social media, and indulge in the occasional television show, but I am intentional and limit the time I spend on these things. Although it's important to stay connected through digital means, it's just as crucial to *unplug* and designate time to focus on the real world. The constant demands of e-mail, texts, and social media can distract us from the immediate—and important—people and tasks in front of us. There is pressure not only to stay connected but also to capture every moment through a camera lens. Unfortunately, this interrupts our connection with the present.

The benefits of unplugging—reduced stress, enhanced creativity, and improved interpersonal connections, to name a few—far outweigh any temporary discomfort. To help you along, I've created a seven-day detox plan to help you unplug. (I am not expecting you to go off the grid!) It's filled with practical steps to help you detox and unplug one task at a time. You may even find that you're able to enjoy the present without pausing to record it.

Wherever you are, be fully there.

- **Day one: turn off push notifications.** Push notifications allow you to receive every new text, e-mail, social media message, and app update on your phone in real time. The moment you get a new message in your inbox, your phone dings. The second someone comments on your social media post, it goes off again. In other words, you are constantly connected unless you turn the notifications off.
- **Day two: unsubscribe from unwanted e-mails.** At the bottom of every e-mail is an option to unsubscribe. This will greatly reduce the number of e-mails you receive. Clear out all that junk e-mail for good. Trust me, you won't miss it.
- **Day three: go out to dinner, and leave your phone at home.** I love doing this. It is so freeing. However, it may be hard for some of you who are so connected to your phone. If you leave your kiddos with a sitter, leave the name of the restaurant where you will be and the phone number, so the sitter can reach you in case of an emergency. This is how we used to do it back in the day.

- **Day four: declutter your devices.** Delete apps you never use from your devices. It will reduce your distractions and make it easier to navigate your phone. Digital clutter is no different from clutter in your home, so clean it up, and get it organized.
- **Day five: set a digital curfew.** Do not check any social media accounts after 6:00 p.m. This includes posting from third-party websites. Not logging on will make it easier to enjoy your evening; not posting reduces the temptation of checking to see how many likes you get.
- **Day six: be fully present.** Whether you are on vacation, out with friends, or sitting at the edge of a waterfall eating a *Bon Appetite*-worthy sandwich, be fully present. Enjoy the moment, without jumping on Instagram to share it. To be fully present, I do a senses exercise. Pick a color, then look around and find everything that is that color. Close your eyes, and listen to all the different sounds that you hear. Take a deep breath, and be mindful of the scents in the air. Touch things around you, like the grass, fabrics, and different textures on different surfaces. (Do not touch people. That is weird.) This is a great way to be in the moment and be present with your body, mind, and spirit.
- **Day seven: read something printed with real ink.** Pick up a paperback instead of a screen. I still to this day do not have any electronic reading device. I love my books. I love the smell of books, and I love to run my fingers through the pages. If you need something to read, visit the library or a local bookstore, and enjoy browsing the shelves. You might find an unexpected surprise.

ONE SIMPLE CHANGE

Unplug the computer, put away the phone, and turn up some good music. Have fun dancing your little heart out! Set aside time to unplug at least once a day, and establish a digital curfew. That sounds simple enough. Your first major challenge will be the appearance of a perfect, beautiful moment. Instead of reaching to snap a picture, experience it with complete attention. Then let it pass. At first, this will feel uncomfortable, but you'll soon realize how wonderful life is when you fully appreciate it in the moment.

CHAPTER 10

SWEAT OFTEN

Do you not know that in a race all the runners run, but
only one receives the prize? So run that you may obtain
it. Every athlete exercises self-control in all things. They
do it to receive a perishable wreath, but we an imperish-
able. So I do not run aimlessly; I do not box as one beat-
ing the air. But I discipline my body and keep it under
control, lest after preaching to others I myself should be
disqualified.

—1 CORINTHIANS 9: 24–27 (ESV)

IF LOSING WEIGHT is your goal, eating right can make your body smaller,
but the only way to reshape, tone, and strengthen your body is through
exercise. The best exercise for this is some form of resistance training
or weight training. If weight loss is your aim, you get the biggest bang
for your buck with this kind of exercise. The more muscle you have, the
faster your metabolism is at rest; therefore, the more energy from fat
your body utilizes. Plus, muscle takes up a lot less room than fat does.
That's why resistance training makes us leaner. The funny thing is that
most people don't understand that muscle weighs more than fat, and
when they look to the scale to measure their progress, they do not like
what they see. It is better to look at your body mass index or the way your
clothes fit you. Go to a trainer or your doctor to get your BMI checked
throughout your training, and mark your progress that way.

Have you ever thought of exercise as food? Well, I have. I believe that many things nourish us. The food we put in our bodies is actually secondary food. Exercise, loving relationships, a fulfilling career, a meaningful spiritual practice, and a connection to our Creator are primary foods. You can eat the perfect diet, but if everything else is suffering, you are not going to experience optimal health and happiness.

Exercise is vital to my mental health, and I am not alone in knowing that. When I exercise my body, breaking a good sweat, all is right in the world. When I exercise, my brain works better. Everything feels better and works better when I exercise. Exercise is the best medicine there is. The scientific evidence demonstrating the positive effects of good nutrition and sleep on stress-induced disorders is good. However, the scientific data on the positive effects of exercise as a treatment method is off the charts. A study conducted in 2005 at Harvard Medical School suggests that using exercise to combat, improve, or even eliminate stress-induced depression and anxiety far outweighs the use of medications to treat the same ailments without exercise. I believe a combination of the two may even be better.

You might be saying, "But I don't like to exercise." In fact, you might just plain hate it. So, what do you do? Well, for most people to incorporate an exercise routine, the routine has to be fun. I am talking about normal people, not the professional athletes and the Arnold Schwarzeneggers of the world who train because they have to. The trick is finding something that keeps you coming back for more.

Find out what motivates you when it comes to physical activity. Do you prefer competition? Joining a sports league can provide you with a healthy outlet, a team dynamic, and a full schedule of games. Do you like to be social and enjoy camaraderie? Then try group fitness classes through a gym, the local YMCA, or an independent specialty studio. The social aspect of this format will eliminate boredom and keep you coming back. Do you prefer to work out alone or one-on-one? Get a basic gym membership that gives you access to a range of equipment. On days you want a buddy, try working with a personal trainer who can also bring some variety to your routine. A trainer can also give you the extra accountability you need to get through the hardest part of any workout—getting dressed and showing up! What if you don't have money for a gym membership or training sessions? There are tons of free exercise apps you can use. They can give you exercises that won't cost a thing and don't require much, if any, equipment. I recommend working up to a goal of exercising for 150 minutes a week. You can break that up a number of ways. For example, you could exercise for five thirty-minute sessions a week. Vary your intensity for the best results and outcome.

Why are you exercising? Is going to the gym five days a week the goal? No. It is a vehicle to get you to your goal. Your goal may be to have more energy to play with your kids or do the things you love. I encourage you to be intentional and really think about why you want to exercise and move your body more. The clearer you are about why you are doing it, the more motivated you will be in achieving that goal. You want to feel good so that you have more energy to do the things you really want to do.

Bonus tip: Some health insurance companies will reward you for moving your body more by helping you track your steps and physical activity. Some even offer discounts on gym memberships. Save some cash by calling your insurance provider and asking about wellness discounts.

GET OUTDOOR EXERCISE

There is an epidemic in America of NDD, or nature-deficit disorder.

—RICHARD LOUV, LAST CHILD IN THE WOODS

There is tremendous nutritional power in the connection between nature and our bodies. Growing up in eastern Washington on my parent's ten-acre farm, I was always outside. Whether it was taking care of the farm by doing my chores, riding my horse in the hills, or just sleeping under the stars, being outside was the natural thing to do. I loved playing outside, and it was hard for my mom to get me to come in for dinner. Today, parents are hard pressed to get a child to want to go outside and play.

Never before in history have children been so plugged in and so out of touch with the natural world. In his book, *Last Child in the Woods*, Richard Louv describes the devastating effects of not connecting with nature on a regular basis. He calls this disconnect nature-deficit disorder, or NDD. As a child advocacy expert, Louv directly links the lack of nature in the lives of today's wired-in generation to some of the most disturbing childhood trends. These trends include the increase in obesity, attention deficit disorder (ADD), and depression. In the book, he describes some startling facts:

> By the 1990s the radius around the home where children were allowed to roam on their own had shrunk to a ninth of what it had been in 1970. Today, average eight-year-olds are better able to identify cartoon characters than native species, such as beetles and oak trees in their own community. The rate at which doctors prescribe antidepressants to children has doubled in the last five years, and recent studies show that too much computer use spells trouble for the developing mind.

He explains that NDD is not a medical condition; it is a description of the costs of alienating humans from nature. This alienation damages children and shapes adults, families, and communities. There are solutions, though, and they are right in our own backyards. In the book, he presents cutting-edge research showing that direct exposure to nature is essential for healthy childhood development—physical, emotional, and spiritual.[7] Louv says, "What's more, nature is a potent

---

7 Richard Louv, *Last Child in the Woods*, (Chapel Hill, North Caroliona, Algonquin Books of Chapel Hill, 2005, 2008) Introduction

therapy for depression, obesity, and ADD. Environmental-based education dramatically improved standardized test scores and grade point average and it develops skills in problem-solving, critical thinking and decision-making. Even creativity is stimulated by childhood experiences in nature."

TAKE VITAMIN D: THE SUNSHINE VITAMIN

I had a scare back in 2010 when I found a suspicious lump in my left breast. Considering I have a family history of breast cancer on both my mother's and my father's sides, I knew it was a cause for concern. Luckily, the lump was just a cyst. The doctors aspirated it and found nothing of concern. I now have routine mammograms.

When I first found the lump and my doctor said it might be cancer, I thought, "No way!" I eat healthy food, exercise, and do everything right. What I know is that cancer is not picky. Anyone can get it—anyone. Look at Lance Armstrong, an elite athlete. My pursuit of optimal health led me to discover the fact that my levels of vitamin D were low. (I am a sunscreen goddess.) Well, less sunscreen and more sun for me now. My vitamin D levels are rising, which is great for my breast health and decreases my chances of getting various forms of cancer. Note that I said "decreases," not "eliminates." The Lord keeps me humble, and for that, I am grateful. Here's to healthy boobies!

What is vitamin D? Vitamin D is necessary for the body to properly absorb calcium and phosphorus—key ingredients for supporting healthy bones and muscles. In the past decade, researchers have discovered that vitamin D also plays an important role in regulating cell growth in the body—including slowing or retarding the growth of many cancer cells. That key unlocked a flood of research into how vitamin D reduces the risk of virtually every form of cancer, heart disease, multiple sclerosis, and many other disorders. Vitamin D comes naturally from exposing our skin to the sun. We get 90 percent of our vitamin D that way.

FIVE BENEFITS TO GETTING SOME SUN!

1. Sunlight profoundly lessens the risk of breast, prostate, colon, and other major cancers.
2. Sunlight dramatically reduces the risk of osteoporosis and hip fractures. This is because the vitamin D we get from sunlight is essential for the absorption of calcium.
3. Sunlight and vitamin D aid in relieving depression and chronic pain.
4. Sunlight and vitamin D help control heart disease and blood pressure.
5. Sunscreens are overused today. As Dr. Marc Sorenson says, they should be used to prevent sunburn but not to block regular sun exposure.

ONE SIMPLE CHANGE

Vitamin D deficiencies are more common now than ever since we are spending more time indoors than we have in the past. The only way to determine your vitamin D levels is to have a blood test. I highly recommend it. Ask your doctor to order the vitamin D 25-hydroxy test (25 OH D). If you come up short, you can solve your problem in just twenty minutes a day. That's all it takes for your body to get the sunlight it needs to make enough vitamin D, even if you're wearing regular summer clothes.

SOAK

I love a good soak in a hot tub or a natural spring, such as Harrison Hot Springs in beautiful British Columbia, Canada. It is one of my favorite places to go to recharge and release all my worries. I particularly enjoy a hot soak in the winter, when it is cold, and after a good workout to soothe my aching muscles. The perfect moment I look forward to is when I first slide down into the warm water. It sends a tingling sensation throughout my entire body, and my relaxation response is quite remarkable. I think, "Ah, there's my happy place." I have found it to be a critical part of my de-stressing regimen, and I highly recommend it.

Natural hot spring retreats have a history of health and healing. Agamemnon, the leader of the Greek armies during the Trojan War, is said to have brought wounded soldiers to Bal Cova Hot Springs near Izmir, Turkey. Even today, the Bal Cova pools are known as the Baths of Agamemnon. Hot springs and saunas work to cleanse and beautify the body by stimulating circulation in the muscles and skin and by increasing internal enzymatic activity.

The skin plays a major role in the eliminative value of hot springs and saunas. We have more than one hundred perspiration glands in a single square centimeter of skin! It is through the pores that up to 30 percent of our body wastes are eliminated. This elimination is greatly stimulated by sweating. Perspiring is necessary not only for our health but also for skin care; it makes skin look beautiful.

Soaking in salty hot spring waters draws oils, fat-soluble toxic materials, and toxic fats out of the skin. Soaking in sulfurous hot spring waters allows the skin to absorb the beauty mineral (sulfur) directly.

Hot spring bathing has been shown to

- improve the skin's suppleness;
- aid in the synthesis of collagen and elastin, thus building elastic connective tissue and erasing wrinkles;
- be loaded with enzymes that scour, clean, and nourish the skin (natural mud baths are particularly loaded with enzymes; in 1956, F. M. Bilyans'kii of the Russian Institute of Biochemistry discovered that the curative properties of muds could be ascribed to the presence of the enzyme catalase);
- help heal acne, eczema, rashes, psoriasis, and other skin challenges; and
- help build strong bones and teeth through the minerals that can be absorbed directly into the body through the skin.

ONE SIMPLE CHANGE

My cheat for a hot spring is to soak in Epsom salts at home. It relieves sore muscles and can also be a great way to detox. I hope you are able to treat yourself to a hot springs retreat in the near future. It is a wonderful gift to your body. Happy soaking!

CHAPTER 11

EAT EMPOWERED

Every moving thing that lives shall be food for you. And
as I gave you the green plants, I give you everything.

—Genesis 9:3 (ESV)

People are fed by the food industry which pays no attention to health, and treated by the health industry which
pays no attention to food.

—Wendell Berry

I BELIEVE THERE are two types of food: primary food and secondary food.
Primary food is the nourishment we receive from our relationships, our
careers, physical activity, and our spiritual practices. Secondary food is
the physical food we place into our bodies. This is what people think of
when they think of nutrition.

Actually, nutrition is about feeding your soul. When you feed your
soul, you are feeding the whole person.

UNDERSTAND PRIMARY FOOD

A scientific experiment that was conducted on laboratory rats illustrates
my point about primary food. The experiment was referred to in a TED
talk called "Everything You Think You Know about Addiction Is Wrong"

by Johann Hari, a journalist who struggled with drug abuse. The purpose of the experiment was to see how environmental factors play into addictive behaviors. The experimenters placed a lone rat in a small, plain cage and gave it the options of drinking water laced with cocaine or drinking plain water. They found that every time the rat went to drink, it always chose the water laced with cocaine. Then they changed the environment. They placed the same rat and the same water options in a large cage with other rats. The cage was filled with an obstacle course, toys, a comfy place to burrow and sleep, and, of course, the stimulation the rat received from the other rats. This time, when the rat drank, it always chose the plain water instead of the water laced with cocaine.

Why do you think this is? It is because the rat's primary food—love, security, and purpose—was being provided. Humans are no different. If you do not have nurturing relationships, if you hate your job, if you have no physical activity, if God feels distant and unknowable, and if your spirit feels dim, how do think you are going to feel? How successful do you think you will be at anything? Your primary food needs are going unmet. Yet people will do what they can to get their needs met, even if that means engaging in destructive behaviors that only provide a temporary fix.

UNDERSTAND SECONDARY FOOD

With so many different dietary theories out there, it is easy to get confused. I am not a food absolutist. What I mean by that is that I do not think there is one way to eat that is right. I believe in finding what works for you, what supports your goals for health and wellness. At different times in my life, including when I was sick, I was very strict about what I ate. I had to be. But I also thought everyone else should eat that way because it was working for me, and I felt amazingly well. I have learned over the years that not only do we have individual food preferences, but our nutritional needs change over time, too. For example, what we needed as a baby is different from what we need as a teenager, as an athlete, during sickness, during pregnancy, and as a senior adult. You get the idea. We spend too much time arguing and raging against everyone's food differences and food discovery journey, and that sort of arguing and raging is not sensible at all. The main thing is we need to eat less crap. I incorporate all the different dietary theories into my coaching. I base each design on the individual and not the theory. I take into consideration your health goals, personal preferences, cultural background, and lifestyle. I believe in the concept of crowding out—adding foods in, rather than taking foods away. When you start incorporating healthier choices, the unhealthy choices naturally get crowded out.

Joshua Rosenthal says, "Given half a chance, the body will heal itself by itself." The point is to give it that chance. But remember that food is only one behavior related to wellness.

UNDERSTAND CRAVINGS

When the diet is wrong, medicine is of no use. When the diet is correct, medicine is of no need.

—AYURVEDIC PROVERB

Anything you put on your body, on your lawn, or on your car you must be willing to eat it. Eventually what you put on your body goes back into the soil, into the earth, and eventually you WILL eat it.

—KIP PASTOR, DIRECTOR OF *IN ORGANIC WE TRUST*

Have you ever wondered why you have food cravings? In terms of primary and secondary foods, what are you satisfied with, and what are you dissatisfied with? Do you have loving, satisfying relationships with family, friends, and your community? Are you satisfied in your career?

Do you have a spiritual practice or relationship with God? Are you getting the proper nutrition from your food, and do you like and enjoy the food you eat? If you are not happy with the primary food in your life and if things are out of balance, that unhappiness and lack of balance can manifest in various ways. To balance the unhappiness, you will try to find a way to feel good and meet your needs. All of us want to feel content and connected to others. But often, we turn to unhealthy lifestyle choices rather than learning how to make the positive changes necessary to have true satisfaction. We create more stress for ourselves instead of creating strategies to combat stress. And if we do not make the necessary, positive changes, we enter into a state of chronic stress. Then the disease process starts.

There are basic dietary and lifestyle recommendations that will help everyone get well, no matter what the disease. Below I've listed the foods to cut back on. Notice that I am not saying you should eliminate these foods from your diet. Just eat less of them.

- Less meat, milk, sugar, and less artificial junk food full of chemicals.
- Less coffee and alcohol. This doesn't mean none—it just means less.
- More fruits, vegetables, and whole foods. Whole foods are foods as close to their original state as possible. The less processed the better.
- Eat organic, humanely raised animal protein or plant-based protein.
- Drink more water.
- Rest and relax.
- Balance primary food.

If meditation seems too hard or too new, you can improve your mood just by eating better. In January 2013, a twenty-one-day study of 281 young adults by Tamlin Connor at the University of Otago in New Zealand discovered a strong relationship between a diet high in fruits and vegetables and a positive mood. According to science, this research is still in its infancy. According to me, it's old news, and science needs to catch up. A long time ago, I knew if I could decode my body, I could figure out a way to overcome the oppressive nature of stress, anxiety, and depression. Years ago, I attended a medical symposium made up of a panel of physicians and scientists. When the Q&A opened to the audience, I quickly raised my hand. I stood before them and asked if there could be a connection between food and mood. Their answer was unequivocally no. They concluded that mood was related to a chemical imbalance or the person had a predisposition for a particular mood, and there was really not much the person could do other than take the available drugs. Food neither contributed to nor prevented mood disorders.

I am grateful for the medications these doctors mentioned, but I have discovered that there is a strong connection between what I put in my body and how it affects my mind, my body, my spirit, and my ability to deal with stress. In particular, too many sugars in the form of refined, processed carbohydrates affect me negatively.

In recent years, doctors and scientists have finally realized that there is a connection between food and mood. There is strong scientific evidence to show that nutrient-dense foods boost the brain's serotonin levels. This could be because these foods are high in antioxidants, which can have a calming effect on all bodily systems. Yes, food changes the chemical balance or imbalance in the brain. I was right all along, and I did not even have to go to medical school. I just needed to listen to my body.

USE PROBIOTICS

Our gut is the powerhouse to our entire endocrine system and our entire immune system. It all starts in the gut. This truth was brought home to me when I was sick. Healing my gut had one of the most profound effects on my overall healing process of everything I did. During that time, I learned so much about my body and the way it works. What an amazing work of art it is! Perfectly created. Fearfully and wonderfully made.

There are different kinds of bacteria in the human digestive system: good bacteria (e.g., probiotics) and bad bacteria (e.g., excess candida yeast). The good bacteria need to outnumber the bad bacteria or the bad bacteria can affect our health in a negative way. Antibiotic use, the wrong foods, and stress are the main culprits in changing the bacteria (also called *flora*) in the digestive tract. Did you know that the bacteria are different in every stage of our digestive system? From mouth to colon, each part has its own little ecosystem, or *microbiome*. When it is not nurtured properly, disease begins.

My doctor put me on a strict diet for three months. For the first month, I could eat only certain things. I eliminated all sugar, including fruit of all kinds; sweeter veggies like beets and carrots; and all grains. I know it sounds very restrictive, but you would be surprised at how much I could eat. I was given a wonderful plan, and I really did not feel deprived. Besides that, I was a highly motivated individual. I wanted healing and would have done anything to become healthier.

After three months, I gradually added foods, learning what worked for my system and what didn't. I had become sensitive to foods I previously had not been sensitive to. Eventually, that sensitivity diminished, but at first I had to be careful about returning to a more normal eating plan.

Together with the restricted diet, the doctor had prescribed high doses of probiotics, which are the good bacteria our bodies need to digest and assimilate the food we eat. Before I sought treatment, I was doing everything right. I was eating good, nutritious food, but because my gut was so messed up, I was not absorbing the nutrients. As a result, I was chronically sick and fatigued, and my weight dropped dramatically. I'm five feet eleven inches tall, and I usually weigh around 145 pounds, but when I was ill, my weight dropped to 123 pounds.

Probiotics have many benefits. They help us regulate metabolism, digest lactose, and modulate the immune system and inflammation.

They also help provide cancer protection and detoxification, improve allergy symptoms by boosting the body's immune system (which increases the body's natural antihistamines), facilitate lipid regulation, function as an antihypertensive, and improve oral health and nutrient utilization.

There are about 3.5 to 4.5 pounds of bacteria in the gut, roughly equal to the total mass of the liver. It's kind of like a little microbrewery.

It amazes me how our digestive system works in perfect harmony when given the right elements. Some of the foods we eat contain parasites, mold, and salmonella, among other things. When the food hits the acid in our stomach, that acid neutralizes almost everything. By the time the food hits our small intestines, there's not a lot of harmful bacteria in there. The next step in digestion is the large intestine, and this is where the magic happens with nutrient absorption and preparation for elimination. Our digestive system takes the good stuff from the food we eat and eliminates the waste. If the right probiotics—the good bacteria—are not present in the large intestine, then waste cannot exit the body in an efficient, timely manner. Trapped inside our bodies, the waste becomes toxic and, if not eliminated, begins the disease process.

As you can see, these little digestive soldiers called probiotics are central to our health and well-being. I could write a whole book on this subject alone.

Hmm. Maybe I will.

I was able to achieve complete healing over the course of two years. However, there was a dramatic improvement in my health after just a few months and a few key lifestyle modifications.

BUY ORGANIC

When it comes to physical food, people often ask me, "Should I eat only organic foods? Is it OK to eat nonorganic? Isn't organic food expensive? What does organic really mean, anyway?"

In answer to the first and second questions, "Should I eat only organic foods? Is it OK to eat nonorganic?" I advise choosing produce according to the buying guide of the so-called *dirty dozen* and *clean fifteen*. This is a good place to start.

Dirty dozen: fruits and veggies that are the most contaminated with pesticides. I recommend that you buy these organic:

- Apples
- Celery
- Tomatoes
- Cucumbers
- Grapes
- Nectarines

- Peaches
- Potatoes
- Spinach
- Strawberries
- Blueberries
- Sweet bell peppers

Green beans and kale are moving up on the most sprayed list, as well.

Clean fifteen: these are the fruits and veggies you can generally buy nonorganic because they are not sprayed as heavily with pesticides:

- Onions
- Avocado
- Sweet corn (watch for GMOs, though)
- Pineapple
- Mango
- Sweet peas
- Eggplant

- Cauliflower
- Asparagus
- Kiwi
- Cabbage
- Watermelon
- Grapefruit
- Sweet potatoes
- Honeydew melon

It is especially important to buy meats and dairy products that are organic or were raised naturally without the use of antibiotics or steroids. Consuming organic food reduces the risk of exposure to pesticide residue and antibiotic resistant bacteria.

In answer to the third question, "Isn't organic food expensive?" I like to point out that buying good-quality food not only saves your body and your mind but also contributes to the health of our earthly environment. If you buy locally grown, in-season produce when possible, you can save money, too. Organic does not have to be cost prohibitive. You can lessen your carbon footprint and find good prices by shopping at farmer's markets, community gardens, and co-ops. Local food requires less packing, preserving, and transporting.

In answer to the last question, "What does organic really mean, anyway?" Organic simply means organic produce and other ingredients are grown without the use of pesticides, synthetic fertilizers, sewage sludge, genetically modified organisms, or ionizing radiation. Animals that produce meat, poultry, eggs, and dairy products do not take antibiotics or growth hormones. It is worth noting that organic does not mean "pesticide free," it means their use is restricted or limited to an allowed list.

The USDA National Organic Program (NOP) defines organic as follows:

> *Organic food is produced by farmers who emphasize the use of renewable resources and the conservation of soil and water to enhance environmental quality for future generations. Organic meat, poultry, eggs, and dairy products come from animals that are given no antibiotics or growth hormones. Organic food is produced without using most conventional pesticides; fertilizers made with synthetic ingredients or sewage sludge; bioengineering; or ionizing radiation. Before a product can be labeled "organic," a Government-approved certifier inspects the farm where the food is grown to make sure the farmer is following all the rules necessary to meet USDA organic standards. Companies that handle or process organic food before it gets to your local supermarket or restaurant must be certified, too.*

These foods are sometimes referred to as *prebiotics*. They are the foods that support and feed the probiotics, setting the stage for optimal health and well-being, by which I mean not only our bodies' health but also that of our minds. Studies have shown that there may be a link between gut health and mental illness. Our digestive system is sometimes referred to as our second brain.

ONE SIMPLE CHANGE

Add a good probiotic to your daily regimen, and eat greens, beans, onions, mushrooms, berries, and seeds—also known as G-BOMBS. Joel Fuhrman is a physician turned cutting-edge natural healer. The first time I heard him speak about his approach to health, nutrition, and healing, I thought my head was going to explode! I was ripe for receiving this information, not only because of my own healing crisis, but also because everything he said made so much sense. The top six foods he recommends you add to your diet are G-BOMBS! So if you are wondering where you should start and what foods you should be eating, consider making Fuhrman's recommendations staples in your everyday diet.

CHAPTER 12

REST AND RELAX

Come with me by yourselves to a quiet place and get
some rest.

—MARK 6:31 (NIV)

Serenity is not freedom from the storm, it is peace
within the storm.

—ANONYMOUS

HERE'S A DEFINITION of resting: to cease work or movement in order to relax, refresh, or recover strength. And here's a definition of relaxing: being at leisure, without tension, anxiety, or urgent demands. In *The Anxiety Cure*, Archibald D. Hart talks about the difference between resting and relaxing. He says that resting is not the same as relaxing. When we are sleeping we may be resting but we are not relaxing. If we are tossing and turning and full of tension, our sleep is not effective. Effective relaxation requires that you not fall asleep. You must remain awake or you do not reap the benefits. We live in a very hurried society, rushing everywhere. We even hurry up to go rest and relax, which makes no sense at all. Life cannot be appreciated when it races past the window of our awareness like a blur.

Often when we are truly resting and relaxing, doing nothing at all, we think we are being weak or lazy. I believe that resting and relaxing are divine activities that display the wisdom of knowing when our bodies need a time-out.

RESTING

[8]Hart reminds us that "a day of rest became mandatory in the laws of the Old Testament. It was called the Sabbath. Any Israelite who violated the Sabbath law paid for this with his or her life. Today, death is still the penalty for not resting. Only now it is a gradual death because the failure to rest aggravates the destructive influence of stress."

The WebMD Anxiety and Panic Disorders Health Center website at www.webmd.com notes that one of the effects of not allowing time for our bodies to recover from the effects of chronic stress is the creation of biologically based anxiety disorders such as panic disorder, social anxiety disorder, specific phobias, and general anxiety disorder.

We feel the need to rest, but our society tells us to stay busy and hurried. Yet the only way to survive the fast pace of modern life is to develop healthy habits that facilitate rest and relaxation. To put it simply, we must rediscover the practice of keeping a Sabbath day of rest. If we want to live a rich, fulfilling life that retains a measure of tranquility, we need a well-honed immune system, a healthy mind, and an abundant supply of natural tranquilizers—all of which we are more likely to have if we consistently take time to rest and make rest one of our priorities.

Real resting takes time: extended, unfrustrated time. Idle time. It also demands that we have nothing waiting in the wings. We have to disconnect, disengage, let go, and forget what we were doing before or what is waiting for us after. We have to separate ourselves from our regular routine, according to Hart.

Time for rest must be taken on a daily basis and not delayed for more than a week. This is the principle of keeping a Sabbath day of rest.

---

8 Archibald D. Hart, *The Anxiety Cure: You Can Find Emotional Tranquility and Wholeness* (Nashville, Tennessee: Thomas Nelson, 1999) 118

Learn what your limitations are, and live within those limitations. If you're pushing yourself to the point of exhaustion, stop and rest. It's like running a marathon. If you keep going at full speed, you're eventually going to collapse. Our bodies give us signals such as fatigue, headache, eyestrain, irritability, and dizziness. Learn to stop before you get to the edge of your limits. Take little breaks throughout the day, week, month, and so on. Taking time for yourself means engaging in pure, luxurious leisure—take time to rediscover yourself, catch up on your feelings, determine new priorities, recreate a sense of balance, and most important of all, restore your soul. This will reconnect you to yourself, to your relationships, and to your Creator.

RELAXING

Relaxation as a treatment modality has been around for years. It increases health and vitality. It lowers stress hormones, including adrenaline, and sadness messengers, like cortisol. It also revs up the immune system, raises tolerance for pain, increases natural tranquilizers, encourages damaged tissue to repair itself, and helps the body to rejuvenate itself. And that's just the short list. It is a powerful method of treating our minds and bodies and preventing fatigue or exhaustion due to stress, and it is a very effective method of alleviating and even eliminating all sorts of conditions. Relaxation is good for everything without exception. That is why you must learn to relax, and you must relax often.

A true relaxation experience does not come from a skeet-shooting competition with your buddies or plopping yourself down in front of the television. Relaxation comes from recognizing where we hold tension in our bodies and finding a way to release that tension. If you take a nice hot bath, a nap, or a stroll through the park on a Sunday afternoon, you're getting the right idea and moving in the right direction.

If true relaxation is what you're looking for, feeling leisurely and unhurried, having no expectations about the outcome of something, and being free to not respond to demands is helpful. In order to counteract stress and anxiety, you must turn off not only your mind but also your muscles. Turning off both turns off the energizing systems in your brain and the adrenal system in your body.

When you experience this very special relaxation response, your adrenaline output drops dramatically, and so does the major chemical culprit that causes stress and anxiety, cortisol. This is why relaxation has such a profound effect on neutralizing anxiety and combating stress.

This drop in adrenaline output is directly related to other beneficial physical changes, such as a decreased heart rate, lower blood pressure, and reduced muscle tension throughout the body. During true relaxation, all muscle pain—including headaches caused by muscle contractions—eases. In addition, the body's metabolic rate slows, reducing wear and tear on the body and even slowing the aging process.

Once your body is in a beneficial state of relaxation, your mind is free to tend to other things. A profound state of relaxation strengthens creative abilities. It strengthens your body's ability to cope with bad stuff, and it unleashes your brainpower to do good, creative stuff.

There is one downside to relaxation. It is hard for some people to do. They may feel that they need to be *productive* and that if they are not being productive, they are being lazy. They might feel uncomfortable doing nothing, so they busy themselves with doing something. I am not saying it is not good to be productive, but rewarding your mind and body with rest is, in actuality, producing tremendous health benefits.

If you have been in a perpetual state of stress, it may take more time for you to tap into your own relaxation response. At first, you might feel quite miserable and experience restlessness, fidgeting, twitching, and a whole lot of wiggling around as you try to find a comfortable position. In fact, when you first begin this practice, you might want to give up. I urge you not to. If you have been in a chronic state of stress, you will go through a withdrawal period. Yes. You will go through withdrawal from stress. Adrenaline is a drug, and you must learn how to come down from it. Trust the process, and don't give up. Small steps lead to great leaps down the path of stress management. Gradually, you will learn how to unwind, and the result will be beautiful: you will feel contentment, peace, serenity, and tranquility. The basic ingredients in all relaxation exercises will get easier the more you practice them.

ONE SIMPLE CHANGE

Relaxation is a wonderful opportunity to connect to your inner self and develop a spiritual practice and habit of self-nurturing. Use that sacred time to pray, meditate, memorize scripture, or just ponder the ways of our marvelous God.

REST AND RELATIONSHIPS

True rest benefits the mind and body, but true rest also has a profound effect on our relationships. In order for our relationships to grow and, more importantly, to thrive, it is essential that we take time for a relationship "rest." During this period, a couple attends to each other. It is important for every couple to find or make the time to be alone together, enjoying each other. One way to do this is to build in time for a special type of rest—the kind that gives priority to rebuilding and strengthening relationships. Failure to observe this type of rest can destroy a marriage as surely as any failure to observe your marital vows, according to Hart.

Resting is not just doing something different from your normal routine. It is not running errands, working out at the gym, or taking an exciting, adventure-filled vacation. On that kind of vacation, there is a daily to-do list, an excursions list, the object of which is to go here and there until we have seen and done it all. If you have ever returned home feeling like you needed a vacation from your vacation, it might be time to reconsider your approach to rest and relaxation.

I went with on an eighth-grade class trip to London and Paris with my daughter and her fifteen classmates. We were there for six days. It was designed to be an exciting, educational adventure that knocked our socks off with each new experience. That mission was accomplished.

Was the trip restful? No. In contrast, I took a kid-free trip to Miami Beach with my husband. Being in that location without any immediate childcare responsibilities put us in a restful state right away. We had unhurried meals, leisurely conversations, and no agenda for our days. We played in the ocean, took naps every day, and took leisurely strolls down the boardwalk. Vacations should leave us feeling rested and renewed, but all too often, they leave us feeling exhausted.

ONE SIMPLE CHANGE

Rest in relationships comes out of presence and availability. Be present with your loved one with no distractions. Make yourself available on a regular basis to be with the one you love. Close relationships require daily connection as well as more long-term attention.

The ten things all relationships need on a regular basis are acceptance, affection, attention, appreciation, approval, comfort, encouragement, respect, support, and security. Be intentional each day while doing something to meet the needs of the ones you love. If you do not nurture your relationships, they suffer greatly.

BIBLIOGRAPHY

Benson, Herbert, and Miriam Z. Klipper. *The Relaxation Response*. New York: HarperCollins, 2009.

Colbert, Don. *Stress Less*. Lake Mary, FL: Siloam, 2005.

Colzato, Lorenza S., Ayka Ozturk, and Bernhard Hommel. "Meditate to Create: The Impact of Focused-Attention and Open-Monitoring Training on Convergent and Divergent Thinking." *Frontiers in Psychology* 3 (2012): 116. Accessed August 29, 2016. http://journal. frontiersin.org/article/10.3389/fpsyg.2012.00116/full.

Douillard, John, DC, CAP. "Nobel Prize Winner Studies Meditation." *LifeSpa*, November 13, 2014. Accessed August 30, 2016. http://lifespa. com/nobel-prize-winner-studies-meditation/.

Environmental Working Group. "Clean Fifteen." Accessed March 8, 2016. https://www.ewg.org/foodnews/clean_fifteen_list.php.

————. "Dirty Dozen." Accessed March 8, 2016. https://www.ewg.org/ foodnews/dirty_dozen_list.php.

Fernandez, Elizabeth. "Meditation Improves Emotional Behaviors in Teachers, Study Finds." *University of California San Francisco News*, March 28, 2012. Accessed August 30, 2016. https://www. ucsf.edu/news/2012/03/11793/meditation-improves-emotional-behaviors-teachers-study-finds.

Hart, Archibald D. "Rest and Relaxation." In *The Anxiety Cure: You Can Find Emotional Tranquility and Wholeness*, 117–29. Nashville, TN: Word Publishing, 1999.

———. "The Anxiety-Depression Connection." In *The Anxiety Cure: You Can Find Emotional Tranquility and Wholeness,* 168. Nashville, TN: Word Publishing, 1999.

Johnson, Sue, PhD. "How to Make Love Last in the Age of Instant Gratification." *MindBodyGreen.* Accessed August 29, 2016. http://www.mindbodygreen.com/revitalize/video/how-to-make-love-last-in-the-age-of-instant-gratification-dr-sue-johnson.

———. *Love Sense: The Revolutionary New Science of Romantic Relationships.* New York: Little, Brown, 2013.

Lemonick, Michael D. "The Power of Mood." *Time,* September 17, 2013.

Louv, Richard. *Last Child in the Woods: Saving Our Children from Nature-Deficit Disorder.* Chapel Hill, NC: Algonquin of Chapel Hill, 2005.

Massage Envy. "Relieve Stress with Massage Therapy." Accessed August 29, 2016. http://www.massageenvy.com/benefits-of-massage-therapy/relieves-stress.aspx.

Miller, Michael Craig, MD. "Exercise and Depression." *Harvard Health.* Accessed August 29, 2016. http://www.health.harvard.edu/mind-and-mood/exercise-and-depression-report-excerpt.

MindBodyGreen. Accessed November 27, 2015. http://www.mindbodygreen.com.

Murphy, Matt. "The Ideal Exercises." *Time,* September 17, 2013.

New York Daily News. "More Fruits and Veggies Can Boost Your Mood." January 25, 2013. http://www.nydailynews.com/life-style/health/fruits-veggies-boost-mood-article-1.1247935.

Orenstein, David. "A Neural Basis for Benefits of Meditation." *Brown University News*, February 13, 2013. Accessed August 30, 2016. https://news.brown.edu/articles/2013/02/mindfulness.

Pastor, Kip. *In Organic We Trust*. DVD. Directed by Kip Pastor. Los Angeles, CA: Pasture Pictures, 2013.

Paul, Sheryl. "How to Have the Greatest Relationship of Your Life." *MindBodyGreen*. Accessed August 29, 2016. http://www.mindbodygreen.com/classes/how-to-have-the-greatest-relationship-of-your-life.

Ragnar, Peter. "Meditation Benefits Shock the Scientific Community." *Natural Health 365*. Accessed August 29, 2016. http://www.naturalhealth365.com/meditation-2.html/.

Rosenthal, Joshua. Bio-individuality course lecture presented at the Institute for Integrative Nutrition, New York, New York, March 2015.

Ryan, Tim. *A Mindful Nation: How a Simple Practice Can Help Us Reduce Stress, Improve Performance, and Recapture the American Spirit*. Carlsbad, CA: Hay House, 2012.

Siegel, Bernie. "How to Use Love as Medicine." Lecture presented at the Institute for Integrative Nutrition, New York, New York, May 2014.

———. "Master the Art of Living." Lecture presented at the Institute for Integrative Nutrition, New York, New York, May 2015.

Sorenson, Marc. "Sunlight and Health." *Natural Health 365*. Accessed March 8, 2016. http://www.naturalhealth365.com/?s=vitamin+D.

Stein, Joel. "Just Say Om." *Time*, August 4, 2003. http://content.time.com/time/magazine/article/0,9171,1005349,00.html.

Szalavitz, Maia. "The Art of Mindfulness Meditation." *Time*, September 17, 2013

Tronick, Edward. "Still Face Experiment." YouTube video, 2:48. Posted November 30, 2009. https://www.youtube.com/watch?v= apzXGEbZht0.

"Organic.org - Organic FAQ." *Organic.org - Organic FAQ*. Foerstel Design, n.d. Web. 07 Sept. 2016. <http://www.organic.org/home/faq>.

Wake Forest Baptist Medical Center. "Researchers Probing Potential Power of Meditation as Therapy." Accessed August 30, 2016. http://www.wakehealth.edu/Neurosciences/Researchers-Probing-Potential-Power-of-Meditation-as-Therapy.htm